practice

pilgrim – yogi – sojourner

practice

KURT KOONTZ

Author of A Million Steps

Practice

ISBN 978-1-7328007-0-0   paperback
ISBN 978-1-000000-0-0   ebook

Cover and Interior Design by:
Chris Treccani
www.3dogcreative.net

Dedication

To Surinder Singh for selflessly sharing yoga.

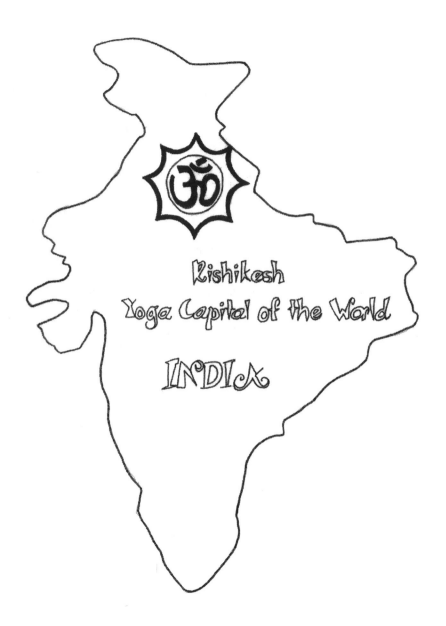

Rishikesh
Yoga Capital of the World

INDIA

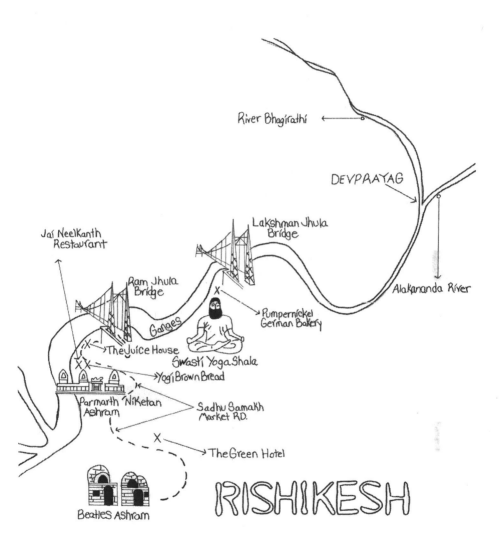

River Bhagirathi ←

DEVPAAYAG

Lakshman Jhula
Bridge

Jai Neelkanth
Restaurant

Ram Jhula
Bridge

Alakananda River

Ganges

X
→ Pumpernickel
German Bakery

X — The Juice House

X
X X
→ Swasti Yoga Shala
→ Yogi Brown Bread

Parmarth Niketan
Ashram

Sadhu Samakh
Market RD.

X
→ The Green Hotel

Beatles Ashram

RISHIKESH

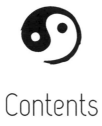

Contents

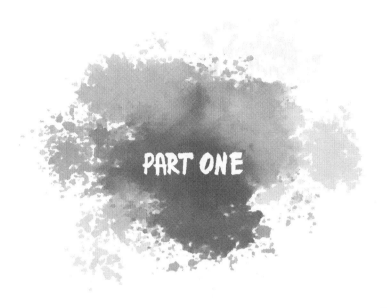

PART ONE

Arrival

After 36 hours of travel, including a nine-hour layover in Delhi, I finally reached my final airport in Dehradun, India. My friend Laurie had arranged for a car to meet me. I scrunched my 6-foot-5 frame into the backseat of a tiny Tata Motors Indica. The driver handed me some chocolate wafers, a bottle of water, and a magazine with stories about my destination—the Parmarth Niketan Ashram in Rishikesh, India.

Everything was fine as we slowly drove to the security gate at the airport. The exit arm rose to mid-windshield level, and then ... the driver slammed the throttle to full force. My left hand found the grab handle, and my right clutched the cracked vinyl seat. We were soon on the right bumper of a truck with "BLOW HORN" painted in big red letters across an enormous green and blue rear. Random chunks of wood filled the payload section while garlands of marigolds swayed alongside metal chains that held the tailgate in place.

Our horn complied with a loud "beep-beep" as we edged into the right lane to pass. Halfway into the maneuver, I saw a lonely scooter with three riders in our path, and I was sure we were going to shatter the bike. Yet, the scooter driver calmly responded with his own "meep-meep" as he edged to his left. My driver threaded the needle between the oncoming cycle and the cargo truck.

For a moment, clarity returned to my head, until I saw something furry run across the road. Two more scampered, following the first. This time I noticed a tail. The next one lunged across on all fours, and I caught a glimpse of a bright red ass as it disappeared into the foliage. In addition to all the honking traffic, this place was crawling with rhesus macaque monkeys.

After about five more minutes of Hollywood stunt-driving techniques, including three-wide on a two-lane road and passing on blind corners, I decided it was time to let go. To preserve my sanity, I divorced fear and assumed the driver valued his life as much as I valued mine. Since I could not mind-drive the car from the backseat, my options were limited to exiting the vehicle or just letting go and enjoying the ride. Thirty minutes of enjoyment later, the car descended a one-lane road to the pinkish stucco walls surrounding the ashram.

My assigned room in the Ganga Block was one of a thousand rooms in the complex. Its 200 square feet included two twin beds, five lights, and a fan. The walls were pale yellow except for an oddly shaped area of about 2 square feet exposing the original mauve wall. Good thing I packed light, as the "closet" was four shelves in a rectangular metal cabinet that wobbled on the slate floor. One hanger draped from the window lock. The bathroom featured a toilet and chronically dripping sink, plus a showerhead sticking out of the wall. The room was so small, the toilet paper had to be removed from the holder to prevent drenching it during the cleansing process.

I wondered, not for the first or the last time, what I was doing here at an "abode dedicated to the welfare of all, lying on the holy banks of Mother

Ganga in the lap of the lush Himalayas." I thought this was just one of my fun solo adventures from my home in Boise, Idaho. I figured I could probably do some yoga as well.

On arrival, it appeared my expectations were far too narrow for the reality of India. This was a lesson I relearned annually on three trips to Rishikesh.

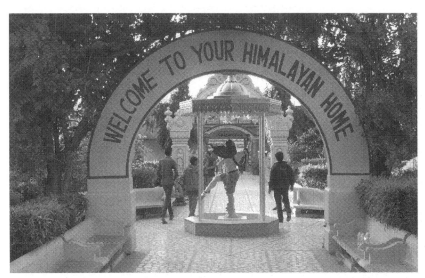

Parmarth Niketan Ashram

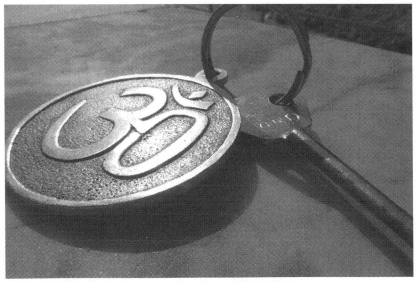

Ashram Room Key

How Did I End Up Here?

That first trip to India, in 2015, was totally unexpected.

I had traveled to many international destinations before, including a nearly 500-mile walk on Spain's El Camino de Santiago in 2012. That trip and the book I wrote about it, *A Million Steps*, subsequently connected me to thousands of new people and places around the world.

In July of 2014, I was invited to speak at the Sun Valley Wellness Festival. One of my perks was a free pass to see the other presentations. Sun Valley provided a very big stage for me, and I was the least important person in a program that included more than 40 speakers. Five of the presenters were *New York Times* bestselling authors who had all appeared on the *Oprah Winfrey Show*.

I was particularly looking forward to hearing Arielle Ford, a celebrated love and relationship expert. I arrived early and began chatting with the man to my right. About halfway through her presentation, Ford introduced her husband in the audience. Guess who was sitting next to me?

After the event, I gave him a copy of my book. One of his friends had walked the famous pilgrimage trail, and he suggested I find her on Facebook. After returning to my room, I searched for her name and was surprised to discover we were already "friends." While writing my first book, I had spent quite a bit of time on Camino-related social media sites where I found interesting people. That is how my friendship began with Laurie Larson.

Just a few months earlier, Laurie had taken a gigantic leap by exiting the traditional workforce and landing in India to become the executive assistant for a prominent spiritual leader. She'd begun to practice Seva, selfless service performed without thought of reward or repayment. During the five to six weeks after Sun Valley, we exchanged a handful of private messages about the Camino and our mutual love for life-changing travel.

Then one day, the conversation shifted. Laurie sent me a short message that said, "I really like Rishikesh and think that you should visit."

I was startled by this communication and didn't know what to make of it. India was not even on my radar. My initial reaction was lukewarm at best.

Later, thinking about Laurie's message, I became more intrigued. I Googled Rishikesh and discovered a city of about 100,000 people in northern India at the base of the Himalayas. The Wikipedia description hooked me on two fronts. First, it described the city as the "Yoga Capital of the World." I had been practicing yoga regularly for about two years at that time. Wikipedia then informed me that in 1968, The Beatles visited the city to learn about Transcendental Meditation at the ashram of Maharishi Mahesh Yogi. Yes, this is where most of the melodies and lyrics were created for *The White Album*.

I began to envision spending a month living in an ashram on the Ganges River. My home for that time would be the largest Hindu ashram in Rishikesh. I suddenly felt a magnetic need to be there and immediately decided to visit. I wanted to lead an intuitive life and have immense trust in my inner-guidance system.

My schedule was wide open, but it took time and patience to get there. I tried to book a flight leaving in a week but found that travel to India required a tourist visa. The questionnaire was complicated. About the only thing they did not demand were the precise dimensions of my most private parts.

I overnighted the documents and began the waiting process. About a week later, I received an email explaining that personal checks were not an accepted form of payment. I was relieved to discover that a Visa card was an appropriate form of payment for a travel visa, and I entered my credit card's digits online.

A few days later, I logged in to the website only to learn that my application was on hold, pending payment. I dialed 1-800-India and navigated through the endless numeric questions in hopes of speaking to a human: press 1 for visa applications, then 1 again for existing applications, another 1 for status updates, and finally, 5 for the San Francisco office. The nice Indian man at the other end of the line informed me that my payment had been received, but I had failed to provide a copy of my receipt. My file would pass to the next step after I sent a physical or electronic copy of my receipt. Laughter filled my head when he told me to download this document from their website and then email it back to them. Every few days afterward, I dialed the magic number and entered 1-1-1-5. About 20 days later, they assured me that there was movement and asked me to call back the next day for confirmation. I followed these instructions exactly but learned that India is closed on the anniversary of Gandhi's birth.

Laurie and I shared many fun messages about this situation. She reminded me that this was an opportunity for her to discover more and broaden the path for my visit. We both knew I would be in India when I was meant to be there. Meanwhile, I was already enjoying the humorous moments in this journey.

Thirty-five days into the visa application process, I received an evening email from the processing company stating that my documents would arrive the next day. I immediately booked a flight departing for Delhi in 36 hours. The next day was oddly normal with some gym time, a yoga class, and lunch with a great friend. Then I mowed the yard, and eventually, packed for the month-long adventure to India. The Camino taught me about packing light, and I used that experience to take no more than I could carry in my rucksack.

While waiting for the plane to depart Boise, I sat next to a couple from India. They were currently living in southern India but had spent 40 years living in Rishikesh, my ultimate destination.

The flights were flawless with 19 hours of actual airtime and layovers in Minneapolis and Paris. The last plane had a nose cam that could be accessed from our seats. Around 11:30 p.m., we began the final descent. When the plane kissed the ground, my screen filled with red, orange, yellow, green, blue, indigo, and violet lights, to represent the seven chakras that energize the body in ancient meditation practices. I was definitely in India.

I had nine more hours to chill in Delhi before flying to Rishikesh. It was my intention to sleep inside the terminal, but my first of many mistakes was to accidentally exit the terminal. I quickly realized that reentry was not an option at that time. A sea of honking taxis, covering four lanes and stretching as far as I could see in both directions, was my welcome mat to the city. Hazy diesel fumes assaulted my eyes and lungs. While trying to get my head around the honking horns, a stranger approached me and said, "Welcome to India. You are in need of help, and I am the one to help you." He proposed a ride to a local hotel where I could get some rest. I was soon raging down a freeway along with another passenger, Francisco from Spain. He had just completed a three-month journey in Nepal and was also on his first visit to India.

Just as our conversation was getting a bit of rhythm, our driver pulled off the freeway and came to a halt on a deserted road. I was sure that my organs would soon be harvested and that my years of travel had finally come to an end. Relief calmed me when I realized this was the switch-a-roo point for Francisco to take a different car headed for another part of the sprawling metropolis. Thirty minutes later, I was standing in the Relaxinn lobby negotiating the terms for my short stay.

However, my sleep there became erratic and pointless. After about five restless hours, I did a quickie tour of Delhi and returned to the airport, headed for Rishikesh.

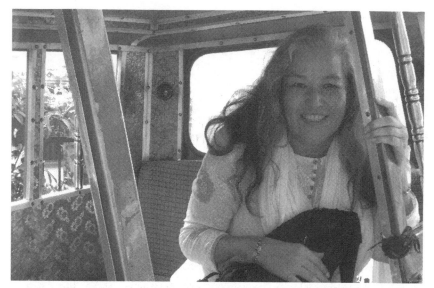

Laurie Larson

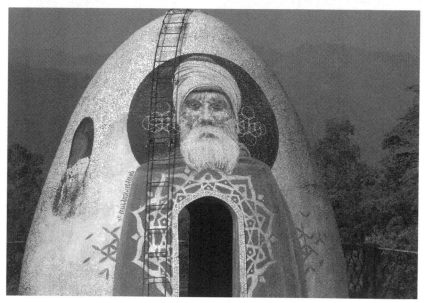

Beatles Ashram Art

First Nights in Rishikesh

On my very first night at the ashram in Rishikesh, I heard young men singing. I looked for the humble, haunting voices and saw ashram students dressed in yellow and orange robes parading through the grounds in two symmetric single-file lines. I followed them to the banks of the Ganges River, where hundreds of people had gathered on the ghat, the steps leading down to the river in front of the ashram. The crowd had come for the Ganga Aarti ceremony that is performed every night of the year on the banks of the Ganges River—Mother Ganga—in Rishikesh.

The riverside celebration began with a fire ceremony or havan, wherein herbs, sweet rice, marigolds, and seeds were offered into the fire pit by 14-16 of the participants surrounding the flames. An elaborate speaker system broadcasted music from the harmonium, the tabla, and tiny hand-held cymbals. While these instruments moved the body, traditional Indian chanting calmed the mind. The ceremony concluded with the lighting of 30-40 large lamps, each with three tiers of multiple burning wicks fueled by ghee. These lamps were passed through the crowd while small puja flower bowls were floated down the river. At the same time, larger burning flames were visible on the other side of the river, at least two football fields away. On that shore, I learned later, bodies were cremated, the ashes returned to Mother Ganga.

That first night I visited Rishikesh, the Austrian ambassador attended Aarti with 15 members of their national symphony. Mozart combined with the harmonium created a peaceful ambience as the political leader poured unifying water from the Danube River into the Ganges. The second night was also a special occasion. Musicians from Israel, Turkey, Ireland, and Saudi Arabia participated in the ceremony. Some say only music can bring the world together. The finale had 1,000 people from every race, color, and creed on their feet singing the following lyrics:

We are one heart.
We are one light.
We are One Source, waking up.
Living one heart. Beaming one light.
Being One Source waking up.
Hallelujah, we are One.
Om Shalom Salam Amen.
Om Shalom Salam Amen.

Afterward, a small group went to satsang where people asked Pujya Swami Chidanand Saraswati (addressed as Swamiji) a question or two. One of the Israeli musicians said that when he is singing, his heart is filled with love. When he is home, his heart is filled with despair for war. The answer, Swamiji said, is to keep singing because it opens the heart to where we become one. As one, we never kill. Bloodshed can only be justified after the lines of separation have been defined.

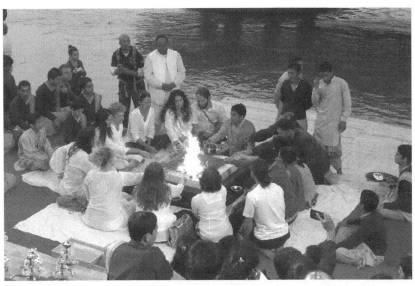

Havan Ceremony

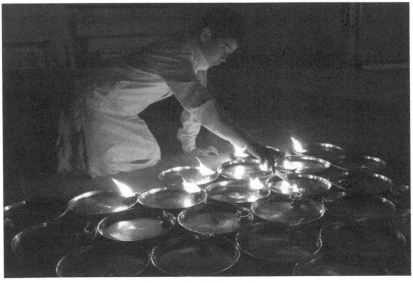

Ganga Aarti Preparation

Narayan's Shop

On my second day in India, I had to take care of business. Laurie promised to take me to a shop where I could buy a local SIM card for my phone.

Yogi's Brown Bread Man Shop is one of many shops along the narrow streets of Rishikesh. The store is about 10 feet wide and maybe 20 feet deep. The many offerings include single cigarettes, yoga mats, soap, hair dye, tampons, peanut butter, biscuits, masala spice, cashews, candy, and phone chips. The owner, Narayan, has occupied this space for 45 years. For the first 25 years, his family lived in the tiny area that is now his office.

Laurie dropped me off, and Narayan invited me into his office to do some phone business. I sat on a piece of plywood that shifted as it met my weight. An old tube TV blared behind my head with Indian politicians hurling insults at each other from the televised floor of Parliament. Shelves covered the walls and were jam-packed with inventory. Narayan took my Samsung phone, removed the back cover, and inserted a new SIM card. For $10, I had a full month of cellular internet as well as unlimited talk and text for all of India. I was pleased to have this task crossed of my list. I bought some cookies and a yoga mat on my way out of the store.

Since this shop was so close to the ashram, I passed it often in the coming weeks. Narayan always greeted me with a warm smile. I never felt that his motives were to get me to buy stuff at his store. He demonstrated genuine interest in my happiness.

One day, he invited me in for India's national drink, chai. Rich black tea is mixed with masala spices and heavy milk to create a warm soulful brew. The mixture is typically served in slender, transparent glass cups. The steamy light brown liquid fills about 3 inches of the cup, leaving just enough room to grasp the cooler rim with a thumb and index finger. (Rookies get burned when they grab the middle.) An invitation to share chai means that the person wants to be a friend.

Instead of recognizing the open arms of this offer, I let fear rule the moment. The only water I drank was either bottled or filtered from the ashram dispensers. I was sure that drinking his tea would be followed by a quick and necessary run to the nearest toilet. I had no idea how offensive it was to rebuff the opportunity to share chai. Each time, his smile remained, but the authenticity of the offer seemed to wane as he narrowed his eyes, seemingly puzzled. I was clueless.

Still, he continued to offer me tea on a daily basis, and after declining 13 times, I finally said yes. We sat in his tiny office, drank his delicious chai, and ate coconut biscuits. It was so enjoyable, I joined him for tea each day until my return to the U.S.

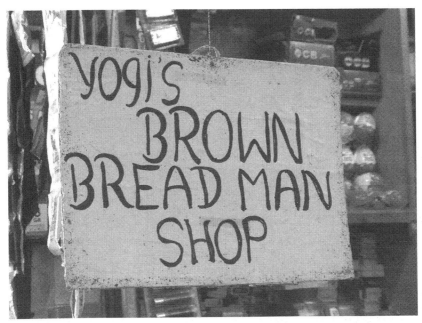

My Second Home

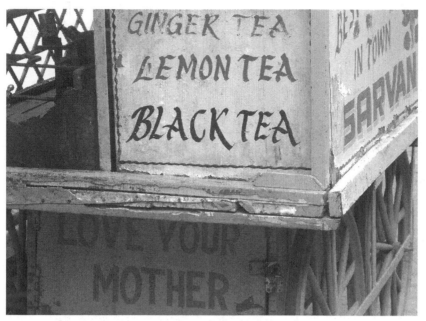

Chai Tea Cart

Vishvas at The Juice House

I was also a regular customer of the The Juice House. The storefront shouts the shop's name with giant red, yellow, blue, and orange letters festooned with garlands of marigolds. The shop's raw materials—limes, mangos, pomegranates, bananas, and pineapples—are stacked high along the street. The constant buzzing of three large blenders can be heard well in advance of arrival. For health and social reasons, this eatery was a favorite spot with the yoga crowd. In addition to amazing smoothies, many people enjoyed the generous portions of fruit salad, muesli, and yogurt curd topped with honey.

Two tables with benches sat three people on either side, but it was very common to see eight people scrunched together at one table. Old, waxy tablecloths made cleanup a breeze from the sticky meals. This place reminded me of the Camino de Santiago, where everyone was welcome at any table. In this case, at both of them. It was also quite common to sit down and find that each person hailed from a different country.

After many visits, I became friends with one of the employees. Vishvas had spent most of his young life in this area. While his actual age was 19, I saw him as an old soul. His kindness and wisdom did not seem to match his youth.

One day I asked him, "Do you do yoga?"

"I have been practicing all my life," he replied. "I am now studying to be a teacher."

"Wow!" I responded. "Where do you teach?"

"I am still studying and not even close to being ready to teach students," he answered. "I have another written test this weekend, and the study is difficult."

A bit surprised, I asked, "How many hours have you accumulated, and when will you be ready?"

"I have 800 hours and need at least 1,000."

In the United States, The Yoga Alliance deems a teacher to be "certified" after 200 hours of training.

By 2018, Vishvas had accumulated 3,500 hours of study.

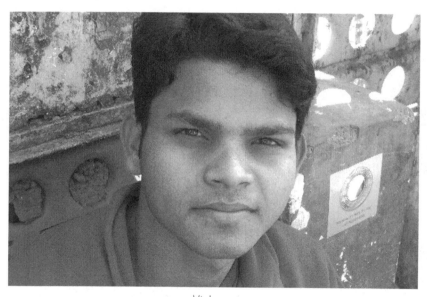

Vishvas

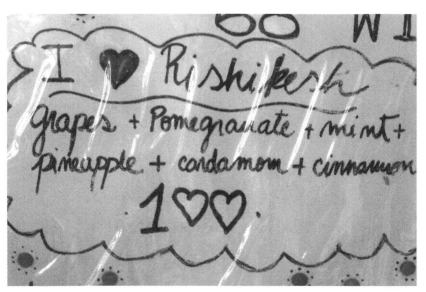

Best Juice Ever

Yoga at the Green Hotel

A few days into my first visit to Rishikesh, I set out to discover the yoga scene. With my camera in hand and yoga mat hanging from my shoulder, I began to wander.

It did not take long to discover signs advertising all types of yoga classes. The sidewalk board for Om Shanti Om highlighted a daily schedule that included Hatha Yoga, Beginner's Yoga, Vinyasa Flow, Meditation, and even Laughter Yoga on Sundays. Just across a small bridge, the World Peace Yoga School featured similar drop-in classes along with 200-hour teacher trainings. I was definitely in the self-professed "Yoga Capital of the World."

Feeling a bit overwhelmed by the choices, I walked to The Juice House to satisfy my nutritional needs. I sat at a community table and began to quiz my fellow travelers about their recommendations for Rishikesh yoga. One friend said, "You will never go wrong with Ashish. He teaches an alignment class at the Green Hotel." Another stated, "If you want strict instruction, cross the river to take a class with Usha Devi at Patanjala Yoga." A third person added, "You should do Surrender Yoga, but take a friend the first time or you will never find the studio. The classes are packed, so go early." I remember thinking about the coolness of the name, Surrender Yoga, and was sure to add this to my short list.

Since the Green Hotel was only a few blocks from my ashram, I decided to make that my target for the next morning. The class was set to begin at 9 a.m. so I arrived at 8:40 to allow for some leeway. After finding the hotel, I was quickly confused and could not locate the famous class.

My lack of Hindi language skills handicapped my ability to communicate with the reception desk workers. Slightly frustrated, I walked out the front door and was then happy to see two young women with yoga mats hanging from their shoulders. I followed them down a short alley that led to a skinny metal staircase. The top of the stairs had barely enough room for one person to stand. When the first lady reached the top, she used some yoga skills to balance on one foot, remove her shoes, and place them on the metal wall rack. I nearly tumbled down the stairs attempting to emulate her performance.

The white marble floor tiles were cold to the feet and helped retain a lower temperature in the room. Piles of yoga mats, boxes filled with straps, mountains of wooden blocks mixed with some foam ones, and bundles of colorful blankets lined the room. Copying a fellow student, I selected a few props and placed a bolster on my mat. Lying on my back, I covered my body with a light blanket and waited for Ashish to arrive. Around 9:15, I broke the silence in the room and asked, "Where is Ashish?" Laughter filled the space and one student responded, "Anything between now and 9:30 is on time for India. You must be new to the area."

Around 9:40, Ashish entered the room, set up his mat, sat down, and dryly said, "Join me in chanting 'OM' three times." He is very focused on alignments and uses straps, chairs, walls, and fellow students as aids to achieve the appropriate postures. This class began with a five-minute flow warm-up followed by Ashish picking a student to demonstrate the downward dog pose. The young lady chosen seemed to be very advanced in her practice. Ashish then dissected her efforts and was quick to identify at least 15 things she was doing wrong. He wanted an arch at the wrist, thigh rotation, toes off the ground and extended.

I was lost. I had no idea that any pose had so many elements. I thought the downward dog meant putting my hands at the top of the mat, feet at the back, and raising my butt to the sky. Toes extended? He must've been joking. After thoroughly kicking her ass, Ashish divided us into groups of three, and we helped each other perform the asana (yoga pose or posture) to the stricter standards. The class continued along similar lines—Ashish selected a guinea pig to model the pose, then we broke into small groups to practice.

About halfway through the class, a young lady grabbed a rope, expertly tied it into wall hooks, and then entered the contraption. With her feet on the wall and the rope supporting her midsection, she hung in place. I casually walked over to ask what she was doing, and she replied, "Stretching my back."

I had never seen a human tethered to a wall. I seemed to be in an alternate universe. In that exact moment, I also saw six monkeys playing on the rooftop, occasionally looking through the glass windows. Feeling like an outsider, I could easily relate to their inquisitive viewpoints.

A few times per week for the rest of my stay, I climbed the metal stairs and practiced yoga at the Green Hotel. The hard exterior of Ashish softened with each lesson, and I found him to be a humorous and loveable teacher. I met so many great people in these classes.

Werner, the German in his mid-60s, wore a biker jacket with a "Masala Rider" logo. His wiry gray hair was contained in a ponytail, and his face was never without an engaging smile.

Chris, a giant man from England, was another regular. He rode to class on his Royal Enfield Classic motorcycle. One day while sipping chai, he told me he'd ridden this bike from the southernmost tip of Goa all the way to the Himalayas. He described the epic journey as being "so many smiles, that my face hurt."

From my Camino experience, I thought I was an expert on packing, but I asked him how he chose for the trip.

He replied, "It must be useful and beautiful."

I thought about this for a moment, then asked, "What is the most useless yet beautiful item you brought on this trip?"

Without hesitation, he said, "My Superman costume."

Several months later, I smiled at a rock music video he posted on his Facebook page, wherein he was featured running down an Indian beach, dressed in his beautiful Superman costume, chased by screaming girls.

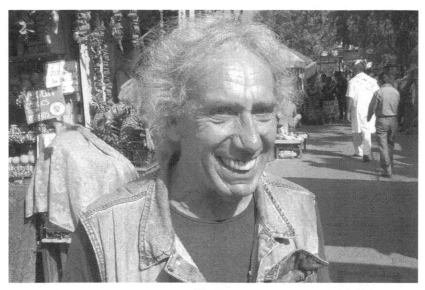

Werner

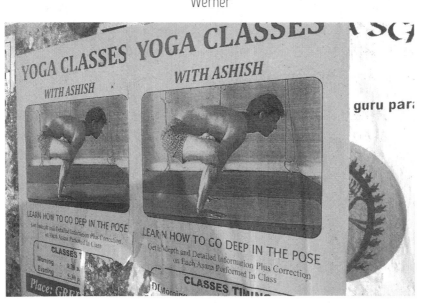

Yoga Ads

The Way to Surrender

One afternoon while enjoying chai with my friend Sharon, she began raving about Surrender Yoga. She reaffirmed the local chatter that this was a good place for practice. She also explained the logistical nightmare of actually locating this yoga studio. At the end of tea, Sharon said, "There is no class now, but let me take you there so you will know the path."

The studio was located only about a mile from Parmarth, but the maze was mind-boggling. From Parmarth, we began walking down Sadhu Samajh Market Road, a narrow street, just 15 feet wide, that separates the ashram from the river ghat. At the first fork, we took a right toward the Chotiwala Restaurant. We turned right at the row of beggars, walked up the hill, took another left at the banyan tree, and kept going toward Punjab National Bank. This next road had several street vendors on one side and permanent benches on the other. Monkeys and locals shared these benches throughout the day. At the next fork, we took a right toward the Hungry Yogi Health Café. Our next turn was a left onto a much smaller road just past a pile of bricks. A right at the next T-intersection then a left past the two-stall, open-air barber shop. We walked in a straight line for a bit, then took another right at another fork. The path narrowed, and the next T-intersection was a dirt path lined with barbed wire on one side. Single file, we walked down the road for about a block, careful not to snag our clothes on the barbs. At the end of the path, we were staring at a five-story black building.

A lone homemade sign was nailed above the doorframe. It was perpendicular to the door and warped slightly toward the ground. Black letters across a white background lined with green on three sides spelled "Swasti Yogshala." I was expecting something like "Swasti Yoga Shala," and the sign was close enough.

Sharon grinned and said, "Well, now you know. Get here early, as there is always a crowd." Then, surprisingly, we took an alternative route back to the ashram. We walked about 10 yards and took our first right to begin an equally confusing maze.

We both laughed at another lonely sign, crooked and torn, hanging above this one-way intersection. It read, "This way to Swasti." (In Hinduism, Swasti refers to "well-being" or "welcome.") In all of Rishikesh, this was the only directional sign that advertised the nearly hidden yoga studio.

The next morning, I woke up early and began the trek to Surrender Yoga. I got lost, of course, but I knew enough about the general location to find my way to the front doors. I arrived at 8 a.m. for the 8:45 drop-in class. Just past the entrance, a large wooden shoe rack appeared to have capacity for at least 50 pairs of sandals. About 15 pairs were already scattered among the five shelves. I walked through the doors and saw not a single person in the lobby, but I heard some chatter from above. I found the staircase and began the ascent.

The second floor had four doors, but no people and no yoga studio. The third floor was identical, but still no people. I followed the voices up one more flight and found about 10 students patiently sitting on the stairs. Some were reading, some were looking at their phones, and others were engaged in hushed conversations. I broke the quiet mood by asking, "Is this Surrender Yoga?"

A young Spanish woman laughingly replied, "It is not Surrender. His name is Surinder. Surinder Singh."

While adjusting to this new, and somewhat disappointing, name-change reality, I sat down and began my wait. The quiet was again broken, but this time the noise emanated from the studio. There must have been a large class in progress as the hallways were suddenly filled with a rich and powerful "OOOOMMMMMMMM," a sound like the vibration of a galactic engine. When the chant subsided, I asked, "What time did that class start? I thought the drop-in was at 8:45."

An Israeli woman looked up from her book and explained, "Surinder does 200-hour teacher trainings. Those people are here for a month-long course."

Our hallway was now quite full, and I could hear voices from the floor below echoing up the stairwell. Mayhem erupted when the fifth-floor studio door opened and those exiting tried to go against the flow of those trying to enter. The incoming class streamed into the studio and rapidly advanced to the pile of yoga mats. People were quick to grab one, locate some empty space and mark their territory. I set up my camp in the back corner of the room.

Bare white walls and a few windows on three sides defined the space. Thin brown carpet lined the floor, and two pillars were oddly located in the middle of the room. Most of the students waited in silence, resting on their mats. I was loving life under my warm blanket, until a fly decided to use my nose as a landing strip.

Every few minutes, another student entered the studio and looked for precious real estate. We crammed closer and closer together to make room. I counted the people in my row and then the number of rows and estimated that the room held about 55 students. Our mats were literally inches apart. When the full room settled down, I closed my eyes again.

Although I heard nothing, the aura in the room suddenly changed. A bit confused, I opened my eyes. I looked toward the front of the room and saw an Indian man seated in the lotus position, his eyes closed in silent meditation. This moment was my first encounter with Surinder.

From this point on, yoga became a transformative practice.

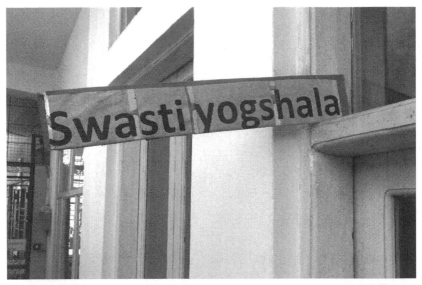

The Yoga Shala

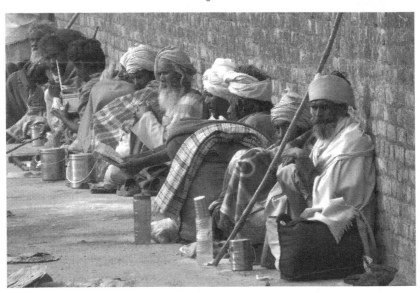

Beggars

Exercise and Yoga

Before India and Surinder, yoga was just another form of exercise and fitness for me. I had a long history of using exercise first as a distraction from my addictions, then as a travel activity. It was, of course, also a way to stay fit and attractive to women.

I had been an active kid who enjoyed skiing and participating in school team sports like football and basketball. When I graduated from high school, my parents gave me a suitcase and a bicycle as graduation gifts. I took both to college.

At the University of Puget Sound, I often used my bike to get away from the noise and stress of being a student. I routinely rode the 15-mile round trip to Point Defiance Park and its scenic loop. I took a stroke at swimming but found it to be very boring. Since I could not see the sweat on my body in the water, I convinced myself there was no way to measure my progress. I tried weightlifting too but found the results slow and the workload heavy.

After graduating from college and going to work at Micron Technology, I found a need for exercise that had very little to do with health. I poured myself into physical fitness to mask my addictions. I convinced myself that I could not possibly have a drinking or smoking problem if I was able to endure strenuous bouts of exercise.

In full-steam mode, I joined a gym and began doing cardio exercise on stationary bikes and stair machines. My sessions were rarely less than an hour. The gym had some racquetball courts and several of the executives were players, so I became one, too. I remember a horrible day when I accidently hit the vice-chairman in the eye with a high-velocity shot. He led the annual shareholder meeting three days later with a gigantic black-and-blue eye.

I also found that group exercise classes were fun. I became a regular in step aerobics classes and a group weightlifting class. The social aspect of exercise was an unexpected benefit.

Two exceptional women worked for me during this time. Since I was the boss, we could often sneak out to the gym during extended lunches for a class or some cardio exercise. As a total jackass, I would smoke on the way to and from the gym. These ladies must have really liked exercise to put up with my ridiculous behavior.

Throughout my 20s, I was in total denial about my addictions. I used my status in the company and my exercise outside the company as blinders to keep my attention off my obvious problems. I operated in this manner throughout that decade.

One day, I tried a new class called Spin. It was a group exercise class taught indoors on stationary bikes. In my early 30s, Spin became my class of choice, and I complemented this activity with some regular weightlifting. Very little of my exercise routine had to do with any kind of inner experience, such as improving my heart or soul, or extending my life. I only worked out for external reasons.

In my mid-30s, when I stopped drinking, I relied on fitness to fill my time in a productive and positive manner. Exercise had become part of my DNA and was something I did at least one hour per day. By this point in my life, I had a wide variety of cardio and weightlifting routines. The Spin classes were fun, but I could never find one that had good and consistent music. To solve the problem, I took a course and became a teacher. The teaching got me back into cycling, which led me to buy a new bike to ride around town. It was sturdy and looked a bit like a mountain bike with skinny tires.

In 2006, I was mowing my yard and saw my neighbor walking to his mailbox. I knew he traveled extensively throughout Europe. At that moment, a crazy idea came to me. My intuitive self, responding to notes from the heart, had sent an urgent travel message. I stopped him and said, "Bob, do you think it would be possible to ride my bike through Europe?"

He grinned and said, "Well, that depends. Do you have the time? Do you have the money? Do you have the guts?"

I nodded yes, finished the yard, and began computer searches on my new crazy idea. Before going to bed, I had booked a round-trip flight to Amsterdam, allowing six weeks to ride across Europe.

Exercise now had new significance in my life, but I was attaching it to a journey without knowing exactly how it fit into the equation. It may have been a crutch for being alone—I could not imagine walking around Europe and taking trains everywhere, but on a bike, I had purpose: a place to leave and a place to go.

I spent all six weeks in motion and rode over 2,000 miles through nine countries. I did not have a map and found tremendous freedom in waking up and letting each day unfold. I came home with a nice feeling of accomplishment. Having survived that experience, I figured I could survive anything. It gave me confidence. The next year, I rode solo from Seattle to San Diego. A year later, my friend Carlos joined me for a two-week ride from Jasper, Alberta to Missoula, Montana.

At the end of that trip, Carlos introduced me to mountain biking. I quickly transitioned to a new form of riding. Also, to satiate my continuing desire for long road bike trips, I began to participate in an annual week-long group ride through Idaho.

Somewhere in my late 40s, I started to experiment with two new group classes at my local gym. The first was classic Pilates. Again, my goal was to get firm abs so women would find me more attractive. My second endeavor was a new class called BodyFlow. It was a 60-minute class that combined Pilates, yoga, and tai chi. I was very attracted to the slow movements and the power required to hold difficult poses.

In 2012, my inner-guidance system engaged again, and I felt the gravitational pull of the Camino de Santiago. I chose the Camino Frances route, which begins at the base of the French Pyrenees Mountains and ends 500 miles later at the famous cathedral in Santiago de Compostela.

I had never considered walking to be a form of exercise, finding the pace ridiculously slow compared to bike riding. I thought it would be hard to cover any appreciable distance in an efficient fashion.

I was so wrong on both fronts. Not only was walking a great form of exercise, it was also easy on the body. The pace of walking and the lack of distractions, like shifting bicycle gears, created the sense of a walking meditation. In the years I raced through countries on a bicycle, I did not realize I had never had time to see the ground below my feet. Which is where life happens.

While walking along the Camino de Santiago, every day was filled with the unknown. I had no idea of the upcoming terrain, no reservations for sleeping, no walking partner, and absolutely no control over the weather. As I let go of my need to control, synchronicity seeped into my life. I began to develop a faith that things would work out. I saw that if someone twisted an ankle on this path, the next pilgrim could easily be an orthopedic surgeon from the Mayo Clinic.

After the Camino, I was very much in tune with the idea of letting go and opening myself up to the unknown. As I tried new things, I also gave up my attachment to the outcome. This attitude led me to my first yoga class.

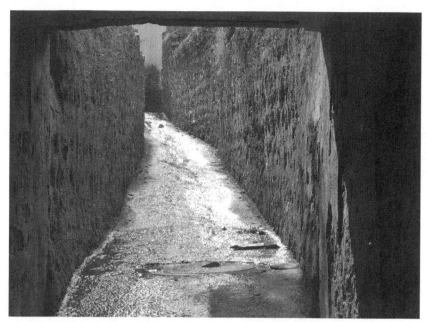

My Path to Yoga

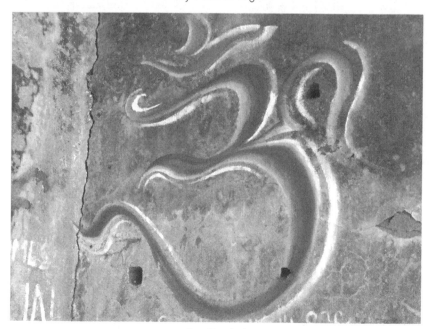

Om Symbol

Hot and Cold Yoga

When I was 48, a few months after I walked the Camino, a good friend invited me to join her at a hot yoga class—a popular class that involves a series of classic asanas (poses) performed in a room heated to 105 degrees and flooded with 40% humidity.

The first thing I noticed was that I was the old guy. Most of the students were very young, very female, and very fit.

I made it through about 30 of the 60 minutes before I felt a need to just lie on my mat and melt into a pool of sweat.

Inspired by the level of difficulty, I formed a habit of taking the class two to three times per week. I was attracted to the challenge of using heat as a new barrier. The heat in itself was something to be respected—I could not just walk in and macho power through.

My local studio in Boise incorporated four "flows" into a class sequence. The flows were fluid movements that were designed to increase the heart rate. These flows also turned on the waterworks, as sweat pooled and soaked into a towel placed on the mat to prevent slipping. The class ended with stretching and the classic shavasana pose.

The heat did increase flexibility, but because I lacked a basic understanding of alignment, it caused me to overstretch in the wrong directions early on. Overall, my body benefited, though initially my lower back experienced some unwanted pain.

I was there for the flexibility of my spine and never imagined the same flexibility could transfer to my mind. About 80% of my classmates were women, and 99% of them were younger than me. Due to the excessive heat and humidity, excess clothing did not exist in these classes. I was sure my social and love life would improve due to participating in this new form of hot exercise. Sad to say, this did not happen.

About one year into my hot practice, I decided to try some cold yoga. I took one class, where we held the poses for a long time, and I immediately knew cold yoga was not for me. My heart rate never rose, and I found no value in just standing in one position. During those classes, I spent more time looking at my watch than at my soul.

My next yoga experience was with Vinyasa yoga in a cool room. This class was much more aligned with my goal of vigorous exercise. The class usually began with stretching that quickly evolved into a series of constant flowing moves. These active movements gave me a sense of accomplishment. During the flow sessions, I also noticed that my mind began to shift into the moment. The moments did not last long, but I had a taste of using yoga to take my mind off yesterday and tomorrow, and into the current moment.

Before traveling to India, I also sampled Yin yoga in beautiful Costa Rica. Yin includes some classic asanas, but the poses are held for longer periods of time and are usually more oriented to stretching than strength. My first Yin class was in an open-air palace covered with a palm-frond thatched roof. The lights were dimmed. Six overhead fans slowly moved the air. Ten candles, in crystal Himalayan holders, flickered throughout the studio. A lone cool cat feigned some interest by lying on the dark hardwood floor. Ocean waves filled the space with a distant, soothing sound.

In this nirvanic atmosphere, my eyes closed, and my breath unexpectedly synchronized with each crashing wave. Then, my interest in the external world ended. I was suspended, as if floating between sleep and consciousness. Prior to that moment, I had found a similar calmness only a few times during relaxing body massages.

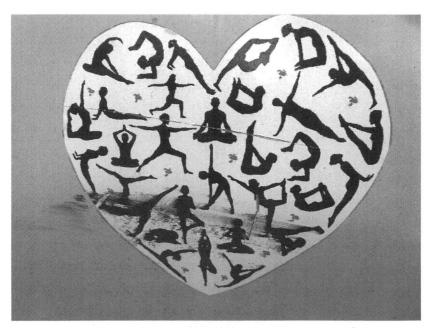

Yoga Love

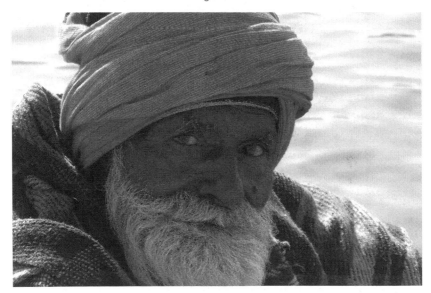

Wisdom

Surinder Yoga

Yoga became a complement to my other exercise routines, although it was still for external reasons like improving flexibility, building core strength, and being around beautiful women. I learned the poses, but the classes were scripted, and there was rarely an explanation of how a pose could take on a deeper meaning at the spiritual level. A yoga session was more like a long exercise class that ended with the teacher saying something about my breath being in your breath. I hoped it wasn't bad breath.

After several years of practice for the wrong reasons, when I found myself in Rishikesh, India, the "Yoga Capital of the World," the first thing I realized was that my head was pretty far up my ass with regard to yoga. On a mechanical basis, most of my poses were horribly flawed. Ashish, my alignment teacher, really helped me surpass the plateaus I had hit in hot yoga. With a little internal or external joint rotation, I was able to engage and control new muscles. I am still not sure where those muscles had been hiding for the previous 50 years.

Later I waded into Surinder's drop-in class, where I made my first real connection to the spiritual side of yoga. In one of my first classes, he said, "Life is very confusing, always moving fast, and most things are very much beyond our control. In yoga, we are able to control the movement, which is the first step to controlling the mind." Suddenly, instead of simply sharing my breath, Surinder had opened entirely new avenues of thought.

Surinder's classes were usually two hours long. The final shavasana was typically 15 minutes and was followed by a short spiritual chat session. To begin the relaxing "corpse pose," he would say, "First scan your body, then make adjustments, and relax into your body." With our eyes closed and our minds falling into a semi-conscious state, Surinder continued, "In your life, when you are in an uncomfortable situation, just make a mental adjustment and relax into the moment." This was my first step in taking yoga off the mat.

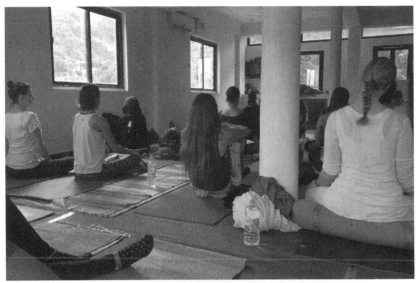

Surinder's Studio

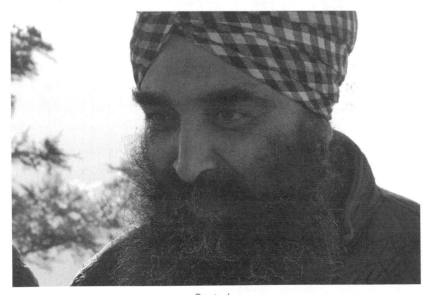

Surinder

Prosthetic Camp

In India, my first lesson was learning to go with the flow—to float through all the doors that opened—while respecting that time had a different meaning in this land. I had no schedule on my first trip to India.

One day, I was eating lunch with my friends Laurie and Vandita in the Parmarth dining hall, making plans to visit another coffee shop, Urban Sip, for chai and chocolate. Laurie received a text inviting us to attend the ashram's prosthetic camp with Swamiji. Minutes later we were walking toward the yoga hall.

I had no idea what to expect from this mini-journey, but as we walked, I thought about the limbless people I regularly saw in India. A few blocks from the ashram, an armless young woman grasped a paintbrush with her toes to create artwork she sold for survival. A legless man used his upper-body strength to propel a crude wooden cart along the dung-infested streets.

At Prosthetic Camp, ashram volunteers used their skills to craft customized arms and legs. Over a three-week period, they had created more than 75 devices, and this final ceremony was to deliver the last 15.

On that emotional day, I watched men, women and children receive the prosthetics that would transform their lives. One particular middle-aged man arrived on homemade crutches. His right leg ended at the knee, the stump rounded like a small grapefruit. He sat down with a fearful face as two ashram volunteers cinched the leather straps to hold the new prosthetic in place. He stood up with the aid of two men and wobbled like a newborn fawn. The men, one under each arm, stabilized him and helped him to a set of parallel bars. I watched as the man clutched the bars with white-knuckled hands and took his first steps in life. Tears streamed down his face and mine as he slowly gained confidence with each small step. That night at Aarti, this man, with a new right leg, proudly left his crutches on the banks for Mother Ganga and vowed to change the world.

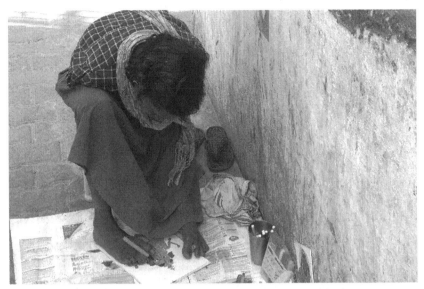

Painting with Toes

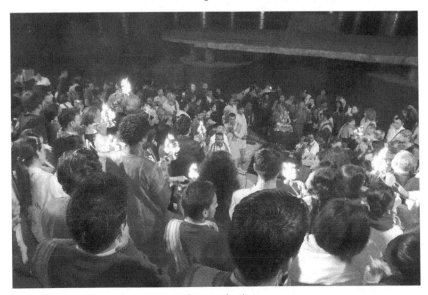

Ganga Aarti

Internal Maps

Each night after the Aarti ceremony, ashram residents were invited to participate in a satsang gathering, where people asked questions of and conversed with the spiritual leader. One night, Swamiji spoke with a group of 20 young adults from Finland. He asked them what they were doing in Rishikesh. One of them replied that their mission was to map the city. Swamiji responded by telling them, that while a worthy cause, they would quickly learn about the locations of the bridges, temples, and restaurants. Most of that knowledge would fade with time.

He encouraged them to spend more effort working on their internal maps. After pulling the obvious weeds and turning the soil, he urged everyone to dig deeper. Using another analogy of the city, he gracefully explained that spiritual people usually avoid the unsavory activity in the dark alleys of Rishikesh. However, on the interior journey, he encouraged us to fully examine the darker alleys, as that is the only way to remove fear with light. The alleys are a grand opportunity, he said, to meet our shadows face to face.

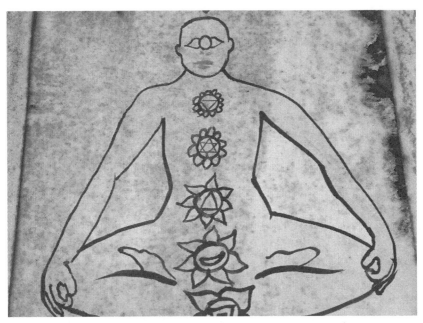

Inside

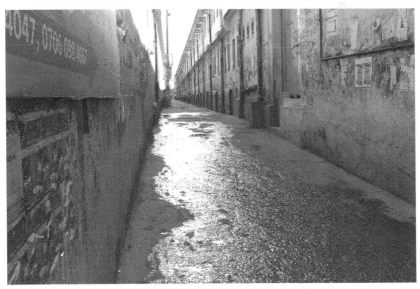

Rishikesh Alley

Pollution

No questions or topics were off-limits at satsang gatherings. One evening an inquisitive man opened with a statement about the beautiful nature of the Indian people. Casting a stereotypical net felt dangerous to me, but I agreed that the physical and spiritual beauty of the Indian population could not be denied.

Unfortunately, while the people exuded beauty, the exterior pollution was obvious and overwhelming. At this time, Delhi was covered in a never-receding cloud of smog, Ganga was the fifth most-polluted river in the world, and nearly half the population had no access to a toilet. During this session of satsang, the perplexed man sought an explanation for the apparent disconnect between such inner beauty and so much pollution.

The leaders quickly acknowledged the external pollution and listed many ongoing efforts to improve the environment. Swamiji, for example, was a co-founder of The Global Interfaith Wash Alliance, which was trying to bring basic sanitation and hygiene to those in need throughout the world. The Alliance was only one of a plethora of projects discussed that evening.

Swamiji suggested that environmental ignorance is rooted in Indian culture because for thousands of years the focus had been inward. Shoes were left outside buildings to prevent the dirt from entering the interior. Negative thoughts were discouraged for the same reason. Hindus believe that we are all part of a universal divine. We don't need to go outside to find the divine because it resides inside every human. Yoga and meditation are methods to strengthen this connection to the inner soul.

Without being offensive, ashram leaders then pointed out the sharp divide between India and the Western World. Beverly Hills, for example, is carpet-bombed with perfectly manicured lawns and ridiculously expensive shiny red Ferraris. Youth is coveted. Porcelain veneers cover teeth, silicone fills breasts and butts, and bling equals status. Balance is the key to life, ashram leaders observed, but Americans seemed to be skewed toward the outward view.

As I listened, I wondered if Western interior pollution rivals the piles of rotting rubbish along the streets of India.

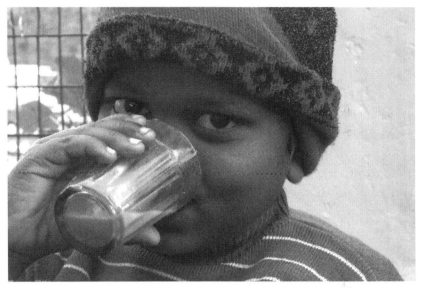

Spiritual Beauty

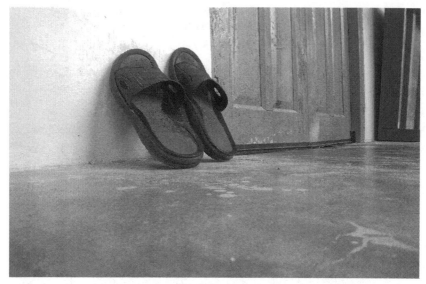

Shoes Outside

Dung Happens

The cow is sacred and deeply respected throughout India. The people of India rely on the cow for milk and dung. The milk is said to have a calming effect, helpful with meditation. Ghee (clarified butter) is burned for fire worship, which is the highest form of prayer for the Hindus. The gentle nature of the cow fits well with the Hindu concept to do no harm to any animal. The dung provides fuel and fertilizer. There is an ample supply!

During one of my first days, I remember sitting in the Honey Hut having a cup of coffee. With its glass doors, the café seemed quite modern. Just as I was recognizing this feeling of Western influence, a cow paused outside the doors to release a fresh pile of dung onto the walkway.

One morning in the ashram, a woman from London quizzed me as I filled my water bottle from the filtration system. She was very concerned that its purity was a farce, and that parasites would attack her system. I assured her that many gallons had traveled through my body without issues, but I could see that my comment did not provide the antidote to her fear.

Later the same day, I saw her again on the main strip by the river. Her eyes were completely fixated on the ground beneath her feet. She was determined to accomplish the impossible task of walking through India without getting cow poo on the shoe.

I have never in my life seen such beauty as the entire scene around Mother Ganga at Rishikesh. Based on water volume, the Ganges is among the largest rivers in the world. She begins the day as a cold gray color that morphs into teal with the first hint of sun. The afternoon rays turn the water into a deep shade of turquoise. Red sunsets cast an orange glow to put the waters to bed. The surface presents as a mesmerizing piece of art, with massive swirls and currents pushing and tugging the waters in divergent paths. The headwaters of the river are tucked nearby in the magnificent Himalayan Mountains that surround the city. Each drop of water travels a relentless 1,569 miles before entering the Bay of Bengal.

I am quite sure my friend from London was so fixated on avoiding the shit that she never had a chance to imbibe the beauty. Dung happens on the streets of India and in our daily lives. Happiness abounds for me when I harmonize with the circumstances and find the beauty in each moment.

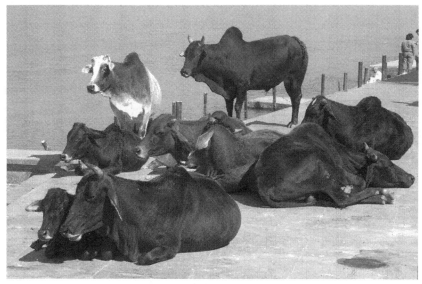

Dung Producers

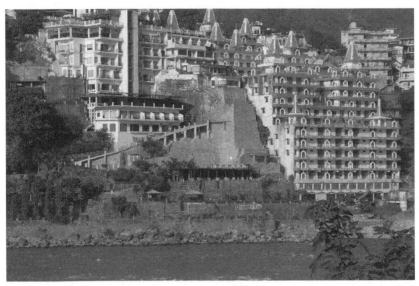

Unlimited Beauty

Street Vendor

Mother Ganga, the heart and soul of Rishikesh, flows mightily through the city. The Sadhu Samajh Market Road follows along the river ghat near the ashram. From dawn to dark, this road is crowded with scooters, pedestrians, cows, and beggars. It is lined on both sides by shops, barber/shave stalls, restaurants, bookstores, fruit carts, street vendors, and even a few coffee shops. The fruit vendors arm themselves with decent-sized wooden sticks to keep the wild monkeys from their banana inventories.

This street became my main path to anything outside the ashram. After a brief time, I could identify my location by the sound of "Shiva Shiva Shambo" broadcasting from the music stalls, the greasy smells from the fried potato vendors, or even the flute music played by a beggar who never changed spots.

At night, the carts were pushed away, the stalls closed, and the stores hidden from view behind metal security shutters. In the morning, the same doors were unlocked and manually hoisted, like sliding garage doors, to the open position. After opening, most store owners used homemade brooms to begin the never-ending task of cleaning the trash and dung that accumulated throughout the night.

On my way to Aarti one evening, a street vendor dressed from head to toe in white looked in my direction and shouted, "Hey, USA!" His interest was in sales, not friendship. His shoulder-strapped tray was loaded with bindi—vials of brilliantly colored kumkuma powders. Hindu people traditionally apply these powders to the center of their foreheads. The colored dots are a religious decoration, representing the third eye of insight and wisdom. The marks are said to strengthen energy and concentration. Surinder would often say, "You have three eyes—two to look and one to see."

This man's tray was filled with packets five wide and at least 20 deep. His wares also included tiny metal stamps with assorted designs. These tools could be dipped into the vials then applied to the forehead. The smaller packets sold for ₹200 (rupees) and the larger ones for ₹500. Within a half-mile, two other men sold the exact same product in the exact same manner. This vendor was lucky to make $15 per day.

Our friendship developed slowly and was hampered by the fact that his fractional ability to speak English was vastly greater than my nonexistent ability to speak Hindi. Occasionally, one of his local friends would sit between us and translate as we enjoyed chai. By then, I had mastered his name, Hoshiyar Singh, but he still called me "USA." I would pass him on the way to yoga, on the way to eat, on the way to Aarti. He always smiled and threw his arms in the air to accompany his "USA" greeting. Sometimes, I bought him breakfast at The Juice House on the way home from yoga class.

One day, he was just wrapping up work and getting on his scooter. He pointed to the back in a manner that meant I was to join him. Not sure of what, why, or where, I hopped on the back. We were soon whizzing through the backroads of Rishikesh. He stopped at a small shop and bought a few apples and one bottle of water. A few moments later, I was entering his home to meet his wife, daughter, and son-in-law.

To be in their home was a surreal experience for me. We sat in a room with one rectangular coffee table, a bed, a couch, and two chairs. His entire family sat on the couch, while I was placed at the other end of the coffee table in a chair. It was almost like an interview. His daughter spoke English, so we were able to communicate as non-stop waves of food piled up on the table.

To his daughter I said, "Please ask your dad if he practices yoga."

I sat amused as the Hindi words flew back and forth. Eventually, she translated his response: "He does practice every single day and all day. His practice is gratitude to be alive, walking by Mother Ganga all day, and meeting people like you."

From that point forward, Hoshiyar stopped referring to me as "USA" and instead used the term "Brother."

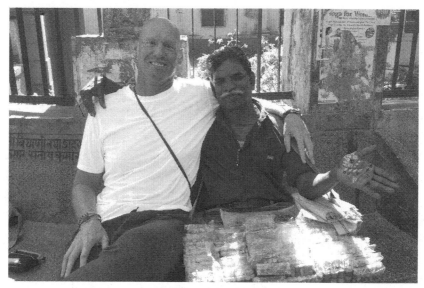

USA and Hoshiyar

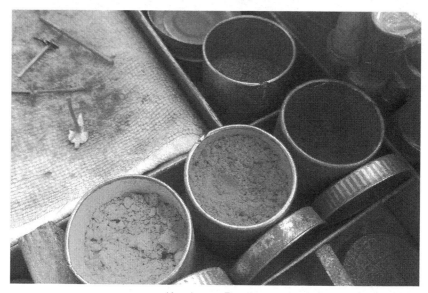

Kumkuma Powder

Journey to Jageshwar

On my fourth night in Rishikesh, as I was having a relaxing dinner with Laurie, one of her co-workers found us and announced, "Great news, there are two seats left for the yoga festival in Jageshwar. Do you want to go?"

It was 8:15 p.m. and the bus was leaving in two hours. The city of Jageshwar was located approximately 200 miles from Rishikesh. In addition to the yoga festival, Jageshwar was known for its 124 stone temples of various sizes, built over 1,100 years ago. This choice was a no-brainer for me. I figured it would take about six hours to get there and the quick journey would be an interesting experience. I went to my room and packed a toothbrush, some undies and socks, a shirt and a light jacket. By 9:15 we were walking 750 feet across the Ram Jhula Bridge.

I was a bit surprised to learn that getting there involved a bus, a train, and another bus. This process seemed like overkill for just a few hundred miles.

I had a lot to learn.

The first cramped bus took us 12 miles from Rishikesh to the Haridwar Train Station, where I had my first experience of the stunning chaos of an Indian train depot. People were sleeping on benches, dirty floors, even the train platforms. Beggars were everywhere and quick to pounce on Westerners.

When I boarded the train, I was happy to hear I had a reserved spot in a sleeper car. Lush images of comfort danced in my mind, then disappeared when I discovered my bed was one of eight in very cramped quarters. The bunks were stacked four high and separated by a 2-foot aisle. Getting into my third-tier bed required some acrobatic contortions. The sheet was like the paper used on a doctor's exam table. My body was too long, so I tried to lie on my side with bent knees. A sudden sit-up in bed was sure to end with my head smashing into the fourth-tier bunk. Eight hours later, we arrived somewhere and boarded a bus. Six hours later, we arrived in Jageshwar.

We had just 20 hours at the yoga festival before we would have to leave again for our return to Rishikesh. The first stop was an amazingly large tent where we watched yoga performances by world-class yogis. Song and dance events alternated with comments given by local dignitaries. I walked through the maze of temples and took an hour-long hike along a scenic nature path.

I asked several times about the sleeping accommodations planned for that night. Each inquiry was met with, "Do not worry, it will all work out." About an hour after dinner and in pitch-black darkness, one of the organizers directed me to go with a small group from the ashram to our rooms. I joined nine students who were enrolled in a month-long yoga-training course at Parmarth. We were driven to The Green River Eco Resort. Six women were assigned to one large room, and four men were assigned to another. There were only two beds, so I looked at my bedmate and said, "Well, I have never slept with a man before, so could you at least tell me your name?" He responded, "Leon. I live in Nairobi and really hope that you do not snore!"

On the return trip, our bus from Jageshwar departed at 1 p.m. to meet a 7:45 p.m. train. Via bus, then train, then bus again, we were scheduled to arrive in Rishikesh at 3 a.m. Laurie woke me up at 2:45 a.m. We got onto the train platform, thinking we were at the right stop to catch the last bus, only to find that another train had derailed. In actuality, our train had stopped due to the derailment and did not move again for four more hours. Eventually, we caught that last bus, but overall, our return trip took 20 hours.

Frustration with the pace would have been the equivalent of resisting the present moment, which, as I was learning, was never a good idea. Instead of whining about the slow speed and cramped quarters, I'm glad I took the opportunity to meet my fellow wanderers and enjoy the Himalayan views. Our group included people from China, Belgium, Hong

Kong, Mexico, England, Kenya, Lithuania, Australia, and Singapore. I was filled with gratitude for the chance to visit this ancient city with these incredible people.

This journey also served as a good reminder to avoid setting rigid expectations, especially when they applied to people, who could be wonderfully spontaneous. A natural unfolding of events would never be in opposition to the rhythm of life.

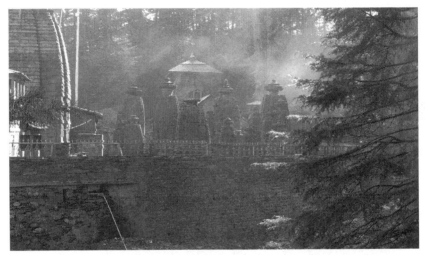

Stone Temples

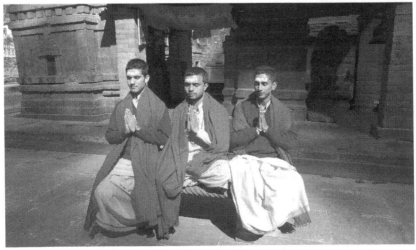

Ashram Students

D.P. Garg

One of the wonders of being open to all experiences is never knowing where the next inspiring chapter will begin or end. On a random Friday, my friend Laurie invited a small group of people to meet with Mr. Garg, a trustee of the ashram. At 4 p.m., I joined a group of five climbing the stairs to his modest second-story room. The entire apartment was probably around 500 square feet.

After Mr. Garg offered us chai and sweets, he asked each of us to tell a bit about our history and the reasons we were visiting Parmarth. He stared intensely into our eyes and heard with his heart as we individually unwove our tangled webs. Mr. Garg, age 88, expressed a deep interest in getting to know us as people, instead of as merely names and faces.

Chiraag, whose name literally meant "lamp, or someone who brings happiness," was first to speak. This 32-year-old man of Indian descent had quit his successful dentistry practice and was taking a year to tour the world in search of a deeper purpose. He had arrived at Parmarth a week earlier from his home in Australia. He had spent the previous day at a local orphanage inspecting (via iPhone) the mouths of 120 children, giving them toothbrushes, followed by a demo on how to use them. His desire to learn and help seemed unstoppable.

Shaochen, a 34-year-old woman from China, followed the Aussie. Without any effort, she radiated love and light. She had left China at the age of 20 and ended up studying at a university in the Netherlands. Until her India trip, she had worked for the government of the Netherlands as an envoy to China. Also in search of a spiritual path, she had scoured the Internet for places in Rishikesh. The Parmarth website slogan, "Do not wait for miracles. You are the miracle," was enough to get her to the banks of Mother Ganga in December. After seven days in Rishikesh, she made the decision to resign her position and devote her life to the service of others. She completed a 30-day yoga training course at the ashram. Following the example of the Hindu god Hanuman, who is believed to have moved the Himalayan Mountains, she declared her intention to save the next generation. Her personal mantra: "There are no boundaries, and we are all one."

Mr. Garg told us how he became a disciple of the original Swamiji at Parmarth in 1950. He came from a privileged family and had a successful business career working for a multinational corporation. Throughout his entire career, he always spent considerable time at the ashram. In 2002, he moved there on a permanent basis to work on special projects for three to four hours a day. His financial capacity would allow him to live the life of luxury sold by Madison Avenue. Instead, he traveled to Bangalore for only a few months of the year and chose to spend the majority of his time at Parmarth. In his tiny apartment, he said, "There is no other place in the world that brings me so much peace."

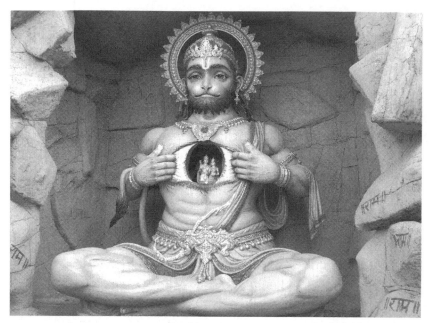

Hanuman

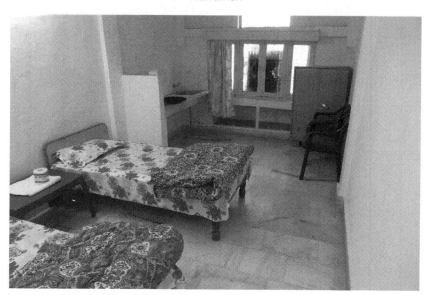

My Ashram Room

Why Solo?

Our visit with Mr. Garg made me explore again the many reasons I love solo travel and adventures.

I am very fortunate that I was able to retire early—and travel often.

I have never been afraid to travel and try something new alone. Adventures with a lover, business partner, or friends and family are always good, but the road less traveled is the solo journey.

My first trip alone was a bit nerve-wracking, with many moments of insecurity. Instead of taking full advantage of my good fortune, I spent time worrying about what other people thought of me. Imagine the level of arrogance it took to think I was important enough to be noticed. Age has taught me to disregard this idiotic thought process.

I now know the big advantages of solo explorations. On my own, I meet people I might not get to know if I were traveling as a pair or with a group. Alone, I also get to choose everything from the destination, wake-up time, and restaurants to the daily list of activities. Each decision is streamlined when solo, while group travel can quickly morph into an exercise in herding cats.

Visiting foreign lands filled with strange customs, languages, and cuisine allows me to see my life with distant eyes. As an outsider, I learn to accept, and survive, everything. That newfound confidence drives out fear and lets in knowledge. For me, building relationships with new people and places provides a perfect classroom for the lessons of life. Travel is a form of therapy that creates a newer and fresher version of me.

When I travel, my surroundings have rarely been as comfortable as my life at home. My budget does not allow for luxurious settings or accommodations. While the first few days in a new place seem abnormal, I soon realize I have more than enough in any given situation. I have slept well in bunks on the Camino, in a cramped and dusty ashram room, and in a tiny rented jungle house in Central America. These experiences serve as a great reminder about the true seeds of happiness. The basis of needing more is a feeling of not having enough. That soil grows only discontentment.

When health issues, financial limitations, or work and family responsibilities keep me close to home, I have found fascinating new worlds and people just around the corner or across town. On the Camino, for example, I set an intention to learn Spanish. Since then, I have spent many hours at my Boise home self-studying with books and online apps. I augment this process by attending classes at a local language school.

I have also remixed my at-home activities to focus on personal growth. Such as, though I enjoy road and mountain biking in Idaho, because I have lived in the state most of my life, some of the trails have become too familiar, too predictable. One day, I woke up and decided to ride each one in the opposite direction. The change in perspective was so simple but required thought and imagination. When confronted with a decision, I always ask myself, "Which one am I most likely to remember five years down the road?" The routine choice is rarely my answer.

Overall, I try to seek solo adventures at the outer edges of my comfort zones. For me, personal growth happens in these unfamiliar territories.

An adventure, either in my neighborhood or in a distant land, gives me something extraordinary to look forward to—an exciting opportunity to open my head and heart to exploring this beautiful world.

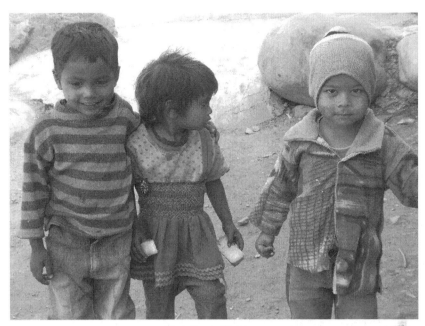

Rishikesh Children

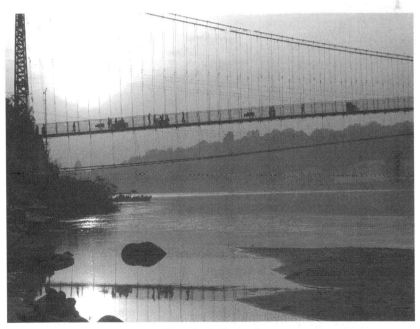

Ram Jhula Sunset

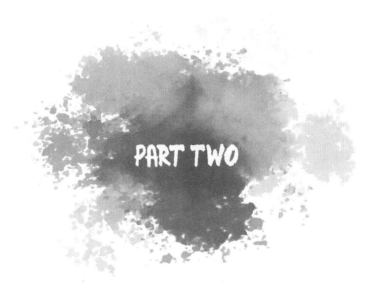

PART TWO

Back to India

When I left India the first time, my rear-view mirror made me feel like I had been on an extended hallucinogenic drug trip. I was there for five weeks of what seemed like constant chaos combined with unfamiliar sounds, scents, foods, and customs. A beautiful trip, but definitely rooted in the surreal, with all of it wrapped in an endless sea of vibrant colors. Rishikesh had been a vast experience, but it was not likely to be a repeat trip, or so I thought.

As the year progressed, I kept having flashbacks to India. It felt like my mind had been on an eating binge and I was now just beginning to digest the thoughts. When I took my annual trip to Palm Springs with my mom, I relived the India experience as I shared my stories with her. I even tried to cook some of the foods I had enjoyed on the banks of Ganga.

After two months in California, I spent a few weeks looking for a yoga-centric community in Central or South America. I chose Montezuma, Costa Rica, hoping to find a yoga scene with deep roots in the spiritual aspects. I wanted to find a method to teach me about taking yoga off the mat and into my life. I was there for a month without encountering anything that compared to India.

As the summer progressed, I continued to drink chai tea and think about the ashram on the banks of the beautiful Ganges River. My heart was telling me to go back to Parmarth and spend at least all of November in Rishikesh.

While planning the return trip to India, I thought about my first and second walks on the Camino in Spain. On my first trip, I had many questions. Could I walk 500 miles? Was sleep possible in bunk beds next to strangers? Could I enjoy walking all day, every day? Well, those questions were answered on the first trip, leaving space in my head and heart to begin the second Camino experience with more room for the unknown. I took that same spirit back to Parmarth for Rishikesh Round Deux.

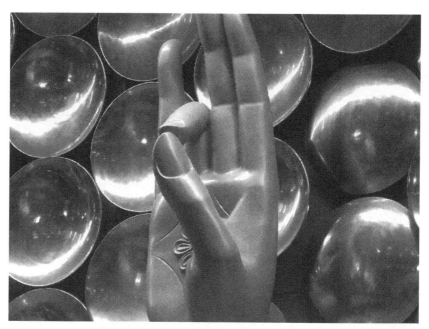

Delhi Airport Art

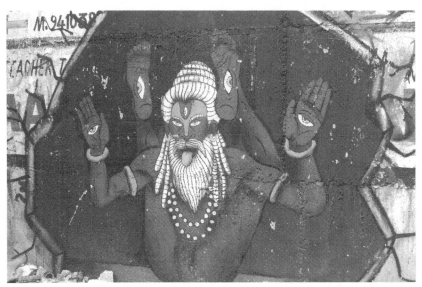

Rishikesh Street Art

Yogi's Brown Bread Man Shop

On my second trip to India, Narayan's shop was among my first stops. His eyes lit up as he instructed his employee Bablu to prepare some chai. We became much better friends over the next five weeks. On most days, I practiced yoga with Surinder in the mornings and then stopped by Narayan's store for chai and biscuits on the way back to the ashram. About two weeks into the trip, he invited me to his home for dinner.

Seven days per week Narayan left his home around 6 a.m., walked a mile to his business, and rarely returned home before 9 p.m. Like many Rishikesh residents, he carried a 4-foot-long wooden club to ward off dogs, monkeys, and even the rare tiger. In the middle of the day, he typically took a bath in Ganga and enjoyed a short nap after lunch at his desk.

On the night of our meal, I met him at the store and he graciously left work very early. He put on his beanie cap, gripped his animal-weapon club, and we began the walk to his home. My first surprise was an immediate diversion to the river, where he said a few words while splashing some water on his face. He explained, "I say goodbye to Ganga every day of my life."

I discovered that I had passed by the brick exterior of Narayan's home many times on the way to yoga class without knowing that this was his residence. He shared the modest home with his wife, three sons, two daughters-in-law, two grandchildren, and four young men who worked at the family businesses. We two ate alone, separate from the rest of his family, in his living room. One of the young workers constantly refilled my plate with chapati, dal, and vegetables. During the meal, Narayan looked and me and said, "I am so envious of your lifestyle. I wish I had a daughter."

I was perplexed by his comment and asked, "How could you not love your existing sons?"

He responded, "Of course I love my sons! But, you do not understand that I will never have the freedom you enjoy. I could never take time and visit foreign lands."

"How does a son prevent you from travel?" I asked.

"My entire life is service to my family," he replied. "The responsibility to a daughter is mainly to educate her and then find her someone to marry. After marriage, she moves out."

I had seen Narayan interact with his three sons, and I had no doubts about his genuine parental love. However, it never entered my mind that the boys did not get their own homes but instead brought their wives and children into the father's household.

Being invited into the home of an Indian person is almost the same as an invitation into the family. Instead of tea with the store owner, I was now having chai with a brother. I was now part of his family.

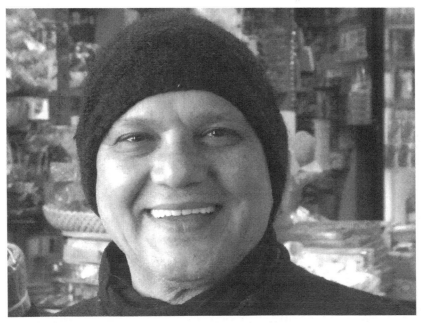

Narayan

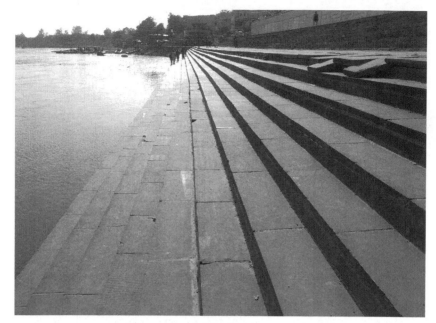

Ghat

Currency Debacle

A person cannot visit India without gaining a better appreciation for the art of patience. Ground transportation is thought to be rapid if the average is above 9 miles per hour over any appreciable distance. Trains that arrive or depart within two hours of the scheduled time are prompt. Yoga classes starting within 15 minutes of the scheduled time are beyond punctual.

My second trip to India, in November of 2016, taught me about patience that went way beyond timeliness.

Upon arrival in Delhi on my second trip, I converted $1,000 in U.S. cash to Indian rupees. That gave me a three-fourth-inch stack of ₹1,000 notes. This amount was more than enough to live like a king for the entire month.

A few days later, I woke up and glanced at my phone. One of the top international stories was about Prime Minister Modi cancelling large denomination currency notes as legal tender. He had announced this decree the previous evening on national TV, and it was effective immediately. "Wow," I thought, "I am so lucky the exchange desk did not give me larger bills." Then I wondered, "What is the biggest rupee note?"

I continued reading the story and found that these big bills were the ₹500 and ₹1,000 notes. At that time, there were five denominations of Indian currency (10, 20, 50, 500, and 1000). The ₹1,000 note is worth about $15. My next thought was, "Well, they must have some type of exchange process. Especially for foreigners. Yes, I am special."

The government ordered the closure of banks and ATMs for two days and planned an archaic program to change existing bills into the new stuff. Foreigners were instructed to visit an airport and convert up to ₹4,000 per day. The round-trip cab fare was ₹2,500, and I was sure there was no way the tiny Dehradun airport had set up a makeshift currency exchange desk. The newspapers estimated that 80% of all transactions in India were cash-based. Very few people had credit cards, and most merchants were not equipped to accept them. That meant that I had ₹250, or $3.30, in spendable Indian money.

The only logical action was to enjoy the day. I started walking to Surinder's yoga class and stopped by Narayan's shop for a cup of chai. He expressed concern about the money issue and had quite a bleak outlook on the government's decision. He felt it was terrible for his family and their businesses. Panicked Indian customers lined up at the store trying to use the banned money. Narayan's son waived them off one by one.

Amid his own business turmoil, Narayan stunned me by saying, "Are you OK? Do you need money? As a guest in my country, it is not acceptable for you to have an unpleasant experience." After an affirmative nod from me, he spoke some Hindi to his son. Moments later, I had ₹1,000 in small denomination bills. Spendable money!

The richness of this moment took a while to marinate. I could hardly believe that my new friend was so genuinely concerned with my wellbeing. "Thank you so much," I said. "I will figure out a way to pay you back." Smiling he said, "That is not your concern. Just make sure to enjoy this day."

The banks eventually reopened with draconian exchange rules. The process reported in the press was obsolete before being implemented. The people without cash to convert faced a similar problem with five-hour waits for ATMs. The machines constantly ran out of money, and withdrawals were limited to ₹1,500 ($20) per day. To exchange money, I waited outside under the relentless Indian sun for three hours. When I finally reached the front of the line, one of three tellers turned me away because I did not have a photocopy of my passport. I had the passport, but they were not in the mood to make a copy.

The next day I was prepared with all appropriate documents, a big bottle of cool water, and a samosa for caloric fuel. While standing in line, I met a young man. He looked at me and said, "Excuse me, sir, you eat at my father's restaurant often. We are so glad to have you as a customer." I responded, "Thank you! What's your name?" He tried to explain about six times, then raised his arm and pointed at his armpit. This is how I met Arpit Gupta.

After four hours in line, I exchanged ₹4,000. At this rate, I would need 16 days and almost 70 hours of spare line time. With a masochistic mindset, I tried for a third day. About two hours into the wait, the line stopped. Without a word, it just ceased moving. I peered into the window and sure enough, both tellers were sitting unencumbered, and the interior of the bank was empty. Wishing for the best, I stayed in line for an additional hour without any movement or hope of progress.

Suddenly, a regular Tata Motors taxi pulled into the road. Four men with machine guns poured out of the bank and approached the dirty white car. The trunk popped open to expose the goods: an actual treasure chest wrapped tight with at least five rusted chains secured with multiple padlocks. I imagined Houdini inside the case as the four guards carried the loot into the bank.

The line resumed. Five hours later, it was my turn. When they entered my passport number into the system, the teller said, "You were here yesterday and must leave. You are only allowed to exchange ₹4,000, one time, at this bank. Next."

That afternoon, I discovered the black market and sold my remaining Indian money for 50% of its value. I paid back Narayan, with interest, immediately.

A few days later and flush with cash, I woke up and went to my tiny bathroom to brush my teeth. When I twisted the water knob, the entire sink fell off the wall. The building was 70 years old and it was just time. The gods must have been looking out for me as it barely missed my toes before shattering on the hard floor. At so early in the morning, nothing could be done, so I did the logical thing: I threw my yoga mat onto my back and began the trek to see my favorite teacher for a morning class.

Surinder, as usual, taught an excellent class, and with such a kind presence. He was gentle and encouraging, a carrier of gratitude. At the end of the class, we pulled our mats close to hear a story. On that day, he discussed our *wants* compared to our actual *needs*.

He said, "You know why nature makes so many good foods? Because that is what you need. You know why nature makes so much beautiful art? Because that is all you need. Nature provides more than you will ever find in an ATM, so today, please enjoy what you have and skip the long bank lines. Practice gratitude by being grateful for what nature has given you."

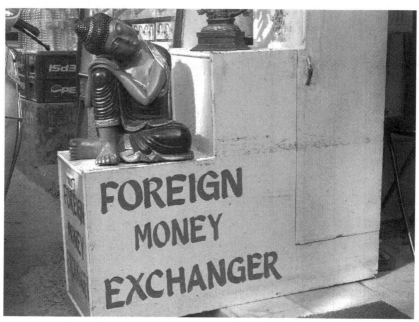

Easy Money

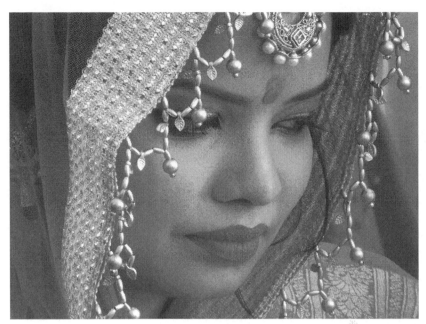

Beautiful Bride

Prana

In my yoga classes, I learned about the power of breath.

On average, the human body will die in approximately three weeks without food, three days without water, and three minutes without oxygen.

In a normal day, we breathe around 20,000 times. In a passive manner, we inhale approximately 500 milliliters of air with each breath. During a long conscious breath, that amount can increase by a factor of seven.

Prana is a Sanskrit word that translates as "vital life force." Prana rides on the breath and is food for the mind and energy for the body. Just like a pen, prana is a tool. Pranayama is a series of breathing exercises that were developed to add consciousness to the breathing process. By controlling the flow of breath, we can increase the amount of prana in the body.

Our breath is the only friend that is with us on the first day, each following day, and our last day. This steadfast friend is always free and never asks for anything in return.

When we focus on the breath, we calm the mind because breath has no demands. The body is the opposite, with endless demands, needs, and desires. Each one tugs on the mind and disturbs the stillness. Through pranayama, we can return the focus inward and onto the breath, resulting in a calm state of mind.

Surinder taught me that a lifelong practice of conscious breathing would lead me to my center.

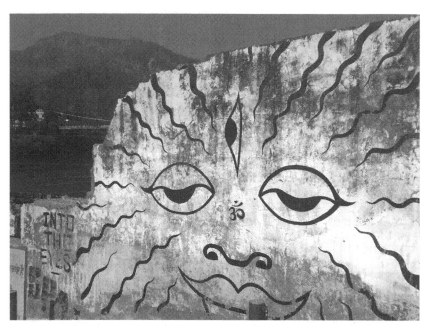

Rishikesh Street Art

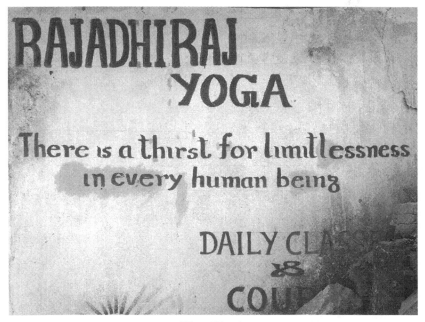

Wise Words

Mango Breath Rebirth

After a random drop-in class with Surinder, my Swedish friends Adam and Anna invited me to their guesthouse for some chai. The short walk from class took us up a small hill to their residence. The communal deck had panoramic views of the valley. While sitting on the soft cushions of a bamboo couch and looking at tiny prayer flags flapping in the wind, Adam said, "We did a rebirthing class last Sunday. Have you ever tried one?"

Thinking they were talking about natural childbirth, I asked, "Are you planning to have a child?"

Anna laughed and answered, "No. Rebirthing is a powerful spiritual exercise. Through specific breathing techniques, you free energy to unlock emotions from your past."

I took a chug of my chai and tried with all my might to hold back a snicker. I am open to many things, but this seemed to be on the edge of my *woo-woo* boundary. After tea, Adam handed me a small folded paper with the details of an upcoming session. I glanced at the paper and placed it in my back pocket.

I had about a mile walk back to the ashram, and I was feeling a bit hungry. I stopped by The Juice House for fruit salad. I took the last open seat at one of the two tables. I recognized two classmates and introduced myself to a few strangers. One was a bald man with stretched earlobe hoops. "Pleased to meet you, Kurt," he replied. "My name is Mango, and I live on the road. My original home is Poland."

"What brings you to Rishikesh?" I asked.

Mango said, "I am here with my love, Natalie. We travel the world and teach a breath rebirthing workshop."

I reached into my pocket and placed Adam's ad on the table.

"How cool," he said. "That is us."

The following Sunday, I walked into the third-floor studio of World Peace Yoga School to be reborn. Sixteen yoga blankets of various colors and Indian designs were interlocked and arranged like an oval racetrack. The cork flooring contrasted with the colorful blankets. Thin blue shades covered the windows. Natural sunlight created a calming blue haze in the room. Two thick pillows were arranged in perfect symmetry on each blanket.

Mango and Natalie were joined by a third teacher named Prema. They sat on three mats at the top of the oval. Prema lit several candles while Natalie ignited a row of handmade incense cones. Smoke trails filled the room with a rich scent.

Mango began by saying, "Welcome to our space. How many people have participated in a rebirthing class?"

Half the class raised their hands in the affirmative. He continued, "Good, this can be an intense experience. I did this the first time at a Rainbow Festival. I ran around camp naked for five hours afterward."

Prema followed up by calmly saying, "This is my passion. Be relaxed and do not become attached to any emotions that arise during the practice. Just experience them."

We began with a 10-minute sequence of five steps. The first was to exaggerate our breathing while flapping our arms and legs freely. The second phase was to express anger by screaming and flexing our bodies. We followed this with two minutes of continuous hopping. The fourth interlude was to freeze and hold any pose. The final physical element was free dance. This combination of erratic movements really did allow a sensation of disconnecting with the past and connecting with the moment.

The instructors then directed us to lie down, close our eyes, and concentrate on our breath. We inhaled with exaggerated chest expansions, and then exhaled by pulling the naval to the spine. The most important part was to make sure there was no pause between the inhale and exhale, making a continuous process with no beginning and no end. The three teachers wandered around the room and individually coached us as we began the deep breaths.

I tried for about three minutes, but nothing was happening. I opened my eyes and saw Prema by my side. She smiled and whispered, "Shhhh," with her index finger pressed against her lips. With her other hand, she gently closed my eyelids and said, "Just continue to breathe. Turn off your mind and take deep breaths. Focus on the air coming in and feel it exit your body."

I followed her gentle instruction and drifted into a hypnotic state of mind. I began to feel an intense tingling in my arms and legs. The sensation literally felt like my blood was flowing through each artery and capillary at an accelerated pace. I continued to drift. With a high-energy flow, random visions from my past flashed into my mind. I followed their instructions and did not dwell on or attach to any of the events. One moment I was reliving my first kiss and the next I was seeing my grandmother's open casket. I just let it flow.

At some point, they asked us to resume natural breathing with pauses between breaths. The tingling sensation ceased, the visions stopped, and I found myself in a very relaxed mood.

I asked Prema, "How long did that last?"

"How long do you think it lasted?" she asked back.

"I am not sure," I replied. "Maybe fifteen minutes?"

She smiled and revealed the truth: "It was almost two hours."

We concluded the session by sharing our experiences with each other. I was not exactly sure what I had let go, but I did have a clean feeling, knowing that some significant life events had been processed. I felt relaxed, and at peace.

Looking back, I often wonder why I use arrogance as a shield of ignorance against the unknown. Stepping into this breathing practice helped me break another barrier to expanding my comfort zones. I have remained in contact with all three teachers, and I am glad our paths crossed in India.

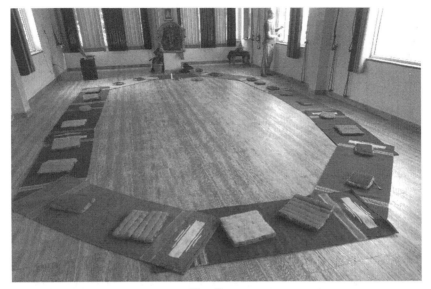

The Room

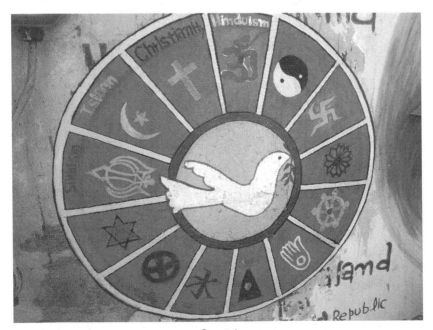

Coexist

Flower Children

The flower sellers of Rishikesh gave me frequent off-the-mat yoga practice on all three of my trips to India.

Early on my first visit, I was in random wandering mode, exploring a new area. I crossed the Ram Jhula Bridge and began walking downstream along the ghat. With my camera in my pocket, I was always looking for unique shots and found an endless supply of subjects.

While strolling along the cracked stairs, I noticed a large pig waddling toward me. The cows and monkeys no longer surprised me, but my first pig was worthy of a snap. I was crouching down for the shot when the animal suddenly scampered in another direction. Apparently, while I was focused on the pig, four young boys had seen an opportunity for commerce. Given my light skin, bald head, towering height, and bright shirts, it would not be unreasonable to say that I stood out in a crowd. They had swarmed me and inadvertently startled the porker.

These adorable boys were half my size and carried cracked plastic colanders loaded with identical inventory. Their foil-lined paper bowls, called puja bowls, were filled with marigolds and topped with flammable waxy cubes resting on quarter-sized ceramic saucers. Each one also included a colorful box of wooden matches and a long stick of incense. Tourists and locals purchased the bowls to ignite the flame, say a prayer, and float their intention down the river.

In unison, the boys began the sales pitch: "Please, please, please, flowers, sir. You want flowers? Please, please, please. Buy flowers, please?"

I had no desire for the flowers but felt a need to reward their relentless efforts. I gave one boy a $10 bill and asked him to share. Instead, he sprinted away and was chased by his three former friends. I later learned that my money could have procured around 40 flower bowls.

On the way back to the bridge, a much less aggressive flower boy approached me. Instead of going for the immediate sale, Ardul was interested in developing a customer. He wanted to know where I lived and what I was doing in India. Then he patiently answered *my* questions about his family and his life. After crossing the bridge together, we prepared to turn in opposite directions. I was headed downstream to the ashram, and he was headed upstream to sell flower bowls. "I really appreciate your being so polite," I told him. "You are now my exclusive supplier of puja bowls." His eyes lit up when I gave him some cash.

During lunch, I asked my friend Laurie how she dealt with the army of children who were selling anything to survive. She said, "I try to persuade them to visit me at the ashram, so I can help enroll them in school."

I became hopeful that I could lead Ardul on a path to school. Each time I bought his flowers, I tried to persuade him to enter the classroom. As far as I know, he still has not done so. But I will be back in Rishikesh soon, and I will continue encouraging Ardul.

On another day, I was lying on a sandy beach by the river. I was dozing off when I felt the presence of another creature. Startled from sleep, I glanced around to find a cow standing just inches from my head. She casually walked past, barely missing my Kindle by half a hoof. I laughed, imagining that call to Amazon customer service.

I covered my eyes with sunglasses and attempted to resume my nap. Before full sleep, I saw a group of flower girls heading in my direction. Three little girls planted their knees inches from my towel, sat down, and stared at me. My lack of motion did not deter their sales pitch. One of the little girls even reached down and removed my sunglasses to see if I had any interest in their flowers.

She said, "I need rupees. Please, please, please, give me some rupees."

Intrigued by the bold intrusion, I shot back, "What if I need rupees? Would you give me some rupees?"

She closed one eye, gave it a thought, and said, "Sir, if you can honestly tell me that you need help, then I will gladly give you my money."

She unzipped her coin purse and tipped the contents onto my towel. They left with all I had.

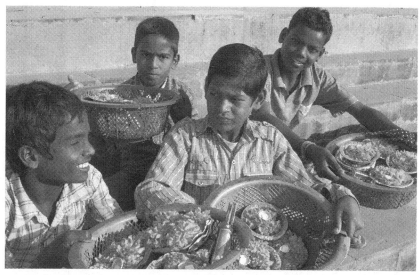

The Boys

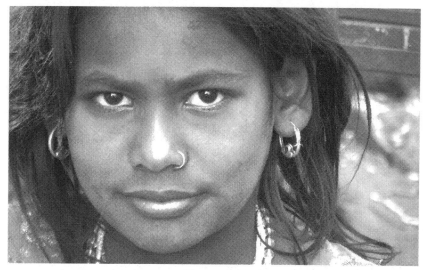

Flower Girl

The Artist

I walked half a mile downstream to visit The Beatles Ashram one day, also during my first visit to India. The 14-acre compound sat on a hill overlooking Mother Ganga.

By 2015, the grounds had been taken over by jungle growth. Dead vines and spider webs covered most of the rock and concrete structures that stood in various states of decay. The only remnant of the former roof in the yoga hall was a lone overhead beam. Local artists had covered many of the surfaces with Beatles-themed murals and song lyrics.

I had spent about an hour wandering around the compound and was preparing to leave when an Indian man approached me with an offer of a tour in exchange for rupees. I paid twice his asking price, which was less than the cost of a latte in a U.S. coffeeshop.

With limited English, he did a nice job of explaining the different buildings and their importance. He guided me through the yoga hall, the meditation domes, the private residences, and the home of Maharishi Mahesh Yogi.

One of the residential buildings had a flat roof topped with a two-story, cone-shaped dome. The interior of the dome was decorated with a colorful abstract representation of Shiva. My guide pointed to the three letters at the bottom of the painting and then pointed to himself. His name was Raj.

I estimated that my new artist friend was in his mid- to late-20s. His face was partially hidden by a goatee beard and mustache. He had a dark green OM symbol tattooed on his neck. He smelled strongly of cannabis, which explained his glossy, dilated eyes. His art was impressive, but he seemed a lost soul.

After the tour we enjoyed some chai at a small stall by the Ganges. He asked for my contact information and then offered transportation services, jungle and temple tours, and rafting trips. He even suggested an excursion to Haridwar.

Later that evening, I received a series of erratic text messages with requests for large sums of money. After repeated calls, I finally answered my phone, only to hear a slurred mess of words. I did not see or hear from Raj again on that trip.

On the first day of my second trip to Rishikesh, I was walking near Parmarth and came across Raj. I approached him from behind as he sat in front of a crude wooden easel. He was adding the final brush strokes to the cheeks of a new tiger painting. I tapped his shoulder and he slowly turned to greet me. It took him a moment, but he widened his smile when he recognized me. His eyes were glazed and his pupils were enormous.

He tried to sell me a painting. I explained that I was there for a month and would not leave India without buying at least one. He then asked me to pay his rent for a month. I did not.

Over the next few weeks, I enjoyed seeing his new works of art. As I got to know him better during our brief visits, I became quite sure that he smoked weed all day to cover some inner wounds. While I still had my own demons, every time I encountered Raj, I was filled with gratitude to be able face them with clear eyes.

Toward the end of the trip, as promised, I purchased a 3-by-2-foot painting from Raj. In this wondrous, Picassoesque painting, traditional vibrant hues are juxtaposed with bold, bending shapes—humans and animals alike seek both purpose and repose. Raj's painting still hangs in my bedroom, a reminder of the power of art to connect us all in our struggles.

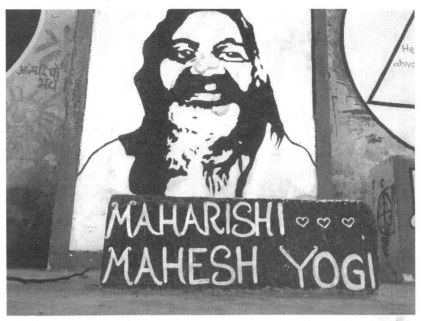

Beatles Ashram Art

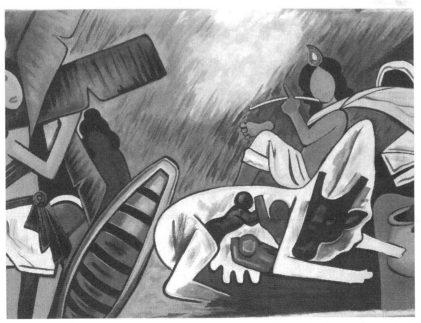

Picassoesque Painting

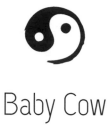

Baby Cow

While walking along the narrow street toward the ashram, I noticed a baby calf draped in burlap, lying on the side of the road. A local Indian man was kneeling and trying to help the ailing animal. Our eyes met as he shook his head in frustration. I could see his mind searching for English words. He finally said, "No power."

The calf was not able to stand and was likely to starve without being able to physically reach a supply of milk. The man lifted the calf, but its legs remained in a twisted fetal pose. He wrapped his arm around the midsection and manually forced each joint into a straight position. It seemed gruesome until I noticed the eager mom moving into position to nurse her baby. The calf was so fresh that its hair was still moist and matted. The man gently guided the calf's mouth to the mom's udder. I felt fortunate to observe the compassion of the stranger combined with the beauty of new life consuming a first meal.

The next night, I walked down the same street and again came across the calf. Someone had placed a multi-colored bead necklace around the tiny animal's neck. Still clad in burlap, the calf seemed to have more strength. I just sat there and gently petted its forehead. The calf seemed to appreciate each stroke. I was so happy that this little creature had survived another day. I continued along my way to the ashram.

The streets of Rishikesh bustled with people and commerce during the day but became bedrooms for beggars and cows during the night. I had been up and down this path so many times that I could recognize almost every beggar at his location. I did give them rupees, but rarely gave them the compassion I felt for the little calf.

The next morning, I was sitting on my perch in Narayan's store. Bablu had just served me tea when a woman came in. Tears streamed from her eyes as she informed Narayan that the calf had not survived the chilly night.

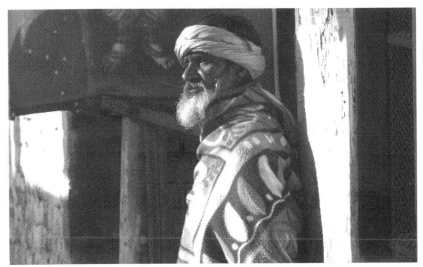

Beautiful Beggar

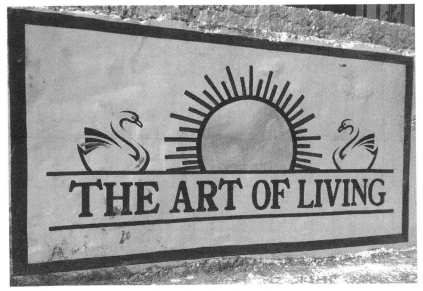

Ravi Shankar Ashram

Self-Compassion

Compassion came naturally to aid a helpless animal. Compassion for an ailing friend or family member, or poor street children, also flowed easily for me. However, compassion for ourselves is just as precious, but rarely practiced. In my yoga practice, I had been learning self-compassion—the art of being totally open to a wound without guarding the heart. With acceptance, my own humanity becomes much more tolerable and allows me to freely embrace others.

Like many people, I think the one person I have abused most in my life is myself. It started with the physical abuse of drugs, tobacco, alcohol, and an unhealthy diet. In addition, an insane voice inside my head delivered massive verbal abuse that never shut up.

Yoga, and especially Surinder, have helped me practice self-compassion by teaching me to accept my limitations in each pose.

The Warrior II asana embodies the spirit of fighting and courage. One day in class I was deep into the pose when Surinder said, "As the destroyer of evil, Shiva was prepared to fight. Learn strength in this pose but accept that the only war that ever needs to be fought is the one that destroys the negative thoughts in your mind."

Now, when I observe my mysterious inner voice that speaks to me without a filter, I try to evaluate the tone from a compassionate perspective. I always ask myself, "Would I ever treat another person in this manner?" The answer is usually no, so I try my best to recognize the words that I just heard, then to rephrase them with love and support, not spite and destruction.

I have come to view this inner voice as a roommate. I have even gone so far as to assign an obnoxious tone to the voice to remind me to be the observer. Having eviction authority over this roommate seems to have fostered a better living relationship.

Humility has also come to me through yoga. Many poses will never happen for me. I am not giving up, just accepting reality. Striving to do the best I can is not the same as pushing through physical pain in a pose.

At 54, there are things that remind me that I am not 24. My metabolism has slowed; unhealthy diet choices quickly show as flab. My skin is wrinkling, and the lines on my forehead are deeper. I had to give up racquetball due to knee injuries. I had to tone back weights for joint issues. Instead of resisting these natural changes and running to the botox store, I dig much deeper and accept myself as is, with unconditional love.

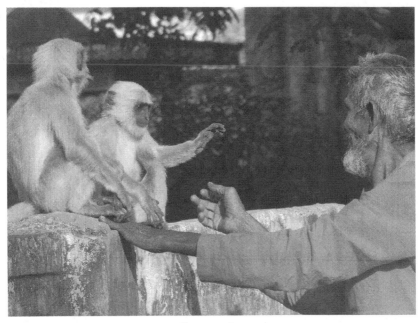

Compassion

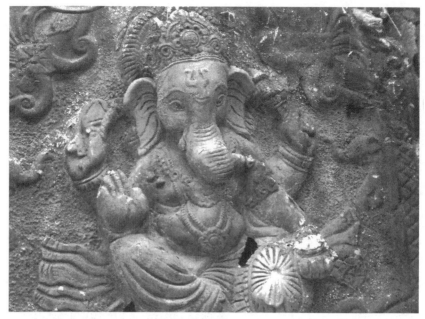

Ganesha

Family Relationships

Accepting my own limitations also helps me accept the limitations of my family relationships.

I am very fortunate to be close to my mom. Every year, we enjoy an annual trip together to Palm Springs, California. Our concentrated time together on these trips allows me to see that our roles are gently shifting. As her mind and body age, these changes require patience on my part and an ability to see things from a different angle.

On the last Palm Springs trip, we bought an extra yoga mat and practiced together a few times per week. Her balance was not great, so most of the poses were seated. I found great pleasure in teaching my mom, a retired teacher, about the spiritual aspects of yoga. When working with her, I also learned more about patience and how to customize yoga for the student. Teaching yoga is not about me showing off some hairy pose, but rather about allowing the student to thrive based on their abilities.

My mom is supportive of my travels but often wonders how I survive and thrive alone. Until recently, she had never been alone, so my solitude seems a mystery to her. I hope that sharing stories of my solo experiences will alleviate her fears.

My brother Nick and I are also close and speak on the phone at least twice per week. He, however, shares not one ounce of my passion for the spiritual path. He thinks it is total bullshit but does not poke fun at me (at least not to my face). In brotherly love, I often remind him that his overactive business career keeps him everywhere but in the moment.

My sister Shawna has no interest in my travel or spiritual journeys whatsoever. In fact, she avoids most contact with me. Yoga has helped me deal with this painful situation as well. In my younger days, I would have thought, "What's wrong with me? Why doesn't my sister like me?" However, yoga has taught me that I control very little beyond the stillness of my own mind and body.

One day during a satsung question-and-answer session, someone asked Surinder, "What do I do with friends and family who have no interest in Dharma?" His answers were typically rather verbose, but this one was like a fist smashing a bug. He said, "You do nothing. They know where you are and will find you when they have interest."

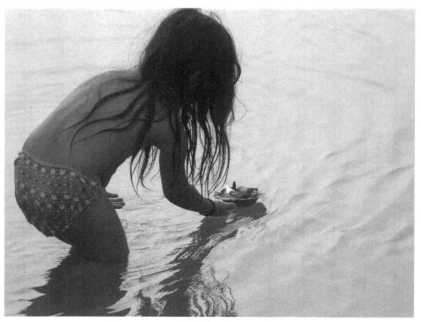

Letting Go

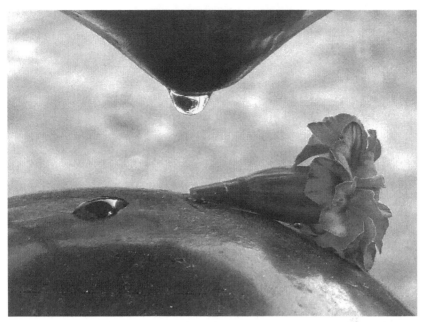

Acceptance

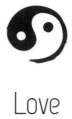

Love

When I was in my early teens, I completely expected to have a life that would include being married and having children. Given my family background, that life would also include a divorce or two.

I do not think that anyone who drinks heavily can have a meaningful romantic relationship, so I was disqualified until my mid-30s. I think I also needed a period of time for me to "wake up and grow up."

Now I sometimes wonder if I use my travel as an excuse to avoid deeply intimate relationships. I am a single guy who has no plans beyond six months and who usually spends six months of the year traveling. Maybe I am hiding behind borders.

Still, I am happy with my life and my lifestyle. I thrive on meeting new people and having new experiences. I do not see myself as half a person just because I do not have a better half. I do not live with the belief that I can complete anyone or that anyone will complete me.

I wake up each day and like to let the day unfold. I accept what happens and try to avoid resisting the present moment. For whatever reason, my love life has not unfolded in a traditional manner. Maybe that is the universe telling me to stay on this path alone.

Love used to be more of a transactional feeling with me—like a business relationship wherein something was surrendered or provided in return for kindness. I now see love as a gift that I can share with anyone. Like a gift, love comes without strings or attachments. I try to spread my version of love freely with all those who cross my path.

Love is wanting the best for everyone and having no attachment to the outcome. Just like success, me winning does not mean you have to lose. Love is not a zero-sum gain. Life offers an infinite and eternal supply of love that is meant to be shared in each interaction.

I used to think that a partner could make me happy, but maturity has taught me that happiness comes from within. Happiness is something to be shared, and not something to be gained from another person.

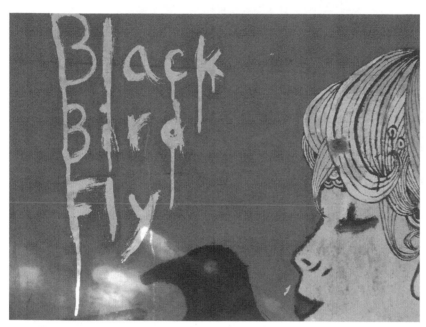

Beatles Ashram Art

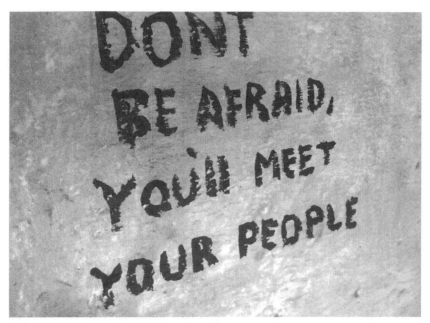

My Motto

Costa Rica Soulful Road

In 2013, when I was writing my first book, I hired a local company to help with the cover design. After reading the manuscript, their creative team came up with four options. It was hard for me to choose, so I posted them on Facebook and decided to let the social-media crowd help with this process.

A new Facebook friend named Soulful Road was quite drawn to one of the images. We exchanged a few private messages about our mutual admiration for the Camino de Santiago. She had already walked the path and was contemplating writing a book about her experience as a pilgrim.

In early 2016, when I was considering my month-long trip to Costa Rica, I noticed several Soulful Road Facebook photos from the country. We resumed our conversation, and she gave me a few recommendations on some spiritually oriented communities and resorts. She also noted from my posts that I had recently been to Rishikesh and expressed an interest in making her first journey to India. I sent her a few links to my blogs with some highlighted stories from that country. As she was preparing to leave Costa Rica, she sent me a photo of a coffee cup adorned with creative monkey art and wrote, "Last coffee before heading out. It all unfolded beautifully. I saved some waves, monkeys, magic for you. Kim." This note was the first time I ever saw her real name. She was heading back to Colorado to be with her ailing mother.

I did visit Montezuma, Costa Rica, and practiced yoga there for the month of May. Although the setting was beautiful, I did not feel much of a spiritual connection to the area. For the first time in my life, I cut a trip short and came home a bit early.

In November of 2016, I was back in Rishikesh and resumed posting many colorful photos on social media. Apparently, India was still deep in Kim Soulful Road's head. She pinged me with a few questions about ashrams and ground transportation. My note said, "I am here for a month and stay at Parmarth Niketan. I do not have a good handle on the guesthouses, but there are many options. I would spin the wheel and book for just a few days. During that time, you can explore and find the correct vibe. Just arrive, wander, and wonder."

In January of 2017, I was feeling the urge to visit a new place, perhaps in Costa Rica. Kim was there in Nosara, so I sent the following message: "Kim, you are a true gem. I am now sure that one day our paths will collide in a really cool manner. I am looking for a place to go for the month of May. My list includes Greece, Sicily, Trinidad, or Costa Rica."

In her reply, Kim sent me a beach photo of a tree with roots exposed from natural erosion of the seawall. The base of the tree was painted white with the number "86" sprayed in a messy blue. Her message said, "On my last morning, I walked down to my favorite spot to give thanks to the big mystery for all of the beauty I'd witnessed during these past few months. On my way in the early morning, a sea turtle had just reached the beach to lay her eggs, a small white butterfly followed me for a while, and I passed a man who was sitting on a giant piece of driftwood playing the ukulele for a one-being audience, his pup. In the spirit of spirit, I have hidden something for you behind #86, up in the roots, just behind the painted part. Maybe it will be there when you are in Nosara in May or it might disappear. Either way, it is all magic."

Although I had not yet decided on a destination for May, Soulful Road Kim already knew the spot.

In May of 2017, I rented "Casita Peace" for a month-long stay in Nosara. This sleepy surfer community had the spiritual and health vibe that was missing from my previous trip to Montezuma. The main beach, Playa Guiones, stretched for 3 miles of soft sand and had a fantastic surf break. Just days after arrival, my routines morphed into enjoying gallo pinto (beans and rice) with eggs and daily yoga classes at Bodhi Tree Yoga or The Harmony Hotel.

On the third day in Nosara, I sent Kim a message asking her for a map to tree #86. She advised me that, if I needed directions, her secret gift was not meant to be found. The next day I was wandering down the beach and noticed the number "19" painted on a beach-side tree. After many more steps, I found tree #20. Given the distance between these two trees, tree #86 was likely to be about 2 miles up the beach.

A light breeze blew as I walked along the smooth sands. Pelicans flew by in groups of three to four, perfectly aligned like drafting bicycle racers. A constant cycle of breaking waves pushed water across the sand. The ebbing water moved random shells that were remixed by the next crashing wave.

I tried to imagine Kim's thoughts when she walked this stretch on her final day in Nosara. Was she thinking about her mom's death? Her next journey? Her purpose?

To arrive at tree #86 felt quite intimate. The roots were exposed in a mazelike manner—wide at the bottom and narrowing on the upward path to the foundation of the tree. At the top point of the roots, the tree's base protected a tiny cave. I reached in and was able to feel something unexpected. My fingers gripped a piece of twine tied to something both smooth and sharp. I pulled on the object and was soon holding Kim's scallop shell from her original walk on the Camino de Santiago—a prized possession for any pilgrim, and hardly an item someone leaves for a Facebook friend.

While I had followed Kim's footsteps to Costa Rica, she had followed mine to India.

After departing Costa Rica, she went straight to Rishikesh for 30 days of satsang with Mooji, a famous spiritual teacher. These spiritual discourse sessions were intended for people to question their purpose at the deepest level. On a random day in March of 2017, I received a solitary photo from Kim. Although the snapshot came with no caption or message, it was immediately familiar to me. It focused on a cardboard sign hanging from thick twine that read, "Yogi's Brown Bread Man Shop." At that time, Kim had no idea of my connection to the store or my dear friend Narayan.

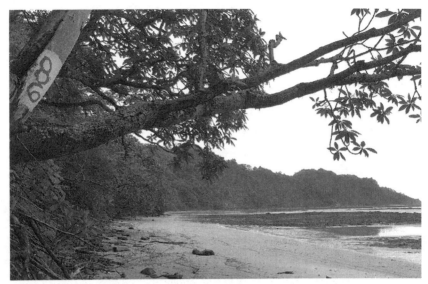

Tree 86

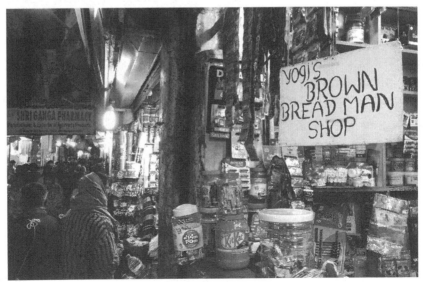

Kim's Photo

Surfing to Restorative Yoga

When in Montezuma in May of 2016, I took surfing lessons from Ricardo a few times per week. By the end of the trip, I was almost a novice, able to stand up on medium-sized waves and ride straight into the shore. No tricks or turns—and with a big emphasis on the word "novice."

On my fifth day in Nosara, I rented a board and set out to advance my surfing skills. Without the slightest idea of where to begin, I cruised the beach with board in hand and looked for instructors teaching beginners. I found my tribe and entered the ocean to master surfing.

I was able to stand about one out of four attempts. After an hour of practice, fatigue set in, and I took a break on the shore. I almost threw in the towel for the day but decided to go back for just a bit more. When I was finally ready to head for shore, two freakish back-to-back waves caught my board. I saw stars as the long board crashed into my head with ridiculous force. For a split second, I thought I had met my end, but I regained my balance. Happy to be alive, I decided to ride a small wave back to the shore. When I lifted my arm to paddle, there was a creepy feeling in my left shoulder, and my upper arm muscle collapsed like a noodle. I knew then that something very bad had happened and that it was likely to change the rest of the month. I left the accident in the water and emerged wondering how it would alter my path.

After a 48-hour love affair with an ice pack, things were not getting better. A Facebook friend introduced me to Cy, a local lady with some mad chiropractic skills. She came to my casita for some adjustments and an hour of massage. She was able to manually move my arm without making me cry. A few days later, another friend introduced me to an experienced physical therapist named Isis. For the remainder of the month, I saw her a few times a week. I was optimistic that a shoulder tendon was simply inflamed, and normal movement would return with rest and time.

After my surfing accident, I tried a Yin class at Bodhi but found the movement too intense for my injured shoulder. I scanned the schedules and discovered something called "restorative yoga." At first, I mistakenly thought this name was just a crafty marketing term for another Yin class, but this new class far exceeded my expectations.

Restorative yoga is a practice that soothes the body and soul by seducing the nervous system into remission. The poses are all done on the floor and usually include pillows and bolsters to support the body. By removing physical stress, mental stress recedes into a dormant state. About every five to ten minutes, the instructor recommends a new position. During the classes, the teachers tend to tell calming stories that encourage deep meditative states.

I spent the entire month enjoying this new form of yoga. One of my favorite teachers, Jane, repeated an invitation I had never heard before. She would say, "Drop in and get to know yourself."

This new endeavor allowed me to learn more about the meditative aspects of yoga and put me in touch with an older group of friends I never would have met in the more active classes.

I came home in June, still in pain, and decided to visit a local shoulder doctor to properly diagnose my problem. I called three places and booked an appointment with the one who could see me the soonest. The meeting with a physician's assistant led me to a pinging tube for an MRI. The nurse said, "You are really lucky to have such a great doctor." I replied, "I didn't know I had a doctor. What's my doctor's name?" That is how I met Dr. Chopp. He advised me to cancel all travel plans for the rest of the year.

Shoulder surgery is not pleasant. I began the recovery process with sleepless nights and bi-weekly physical therapy appointments. Three times a day for over three months, I did different sets of exercises to improve my range of motion. Progress was *so* slow. In September, they gave me the OK to do some light resistance work with weights. Prior to that time, I was restricted to no more than a coffee cup as a bicep curl.

In late October, during a routine follow-up with Dr. Chopp, he said, "Kurt, you are doing well. I may be able to turn you loose on your bike in a few weeks." Quite pleased, I asked about yoga and he said, "Well, maybe in early November."

With a smile, I pressed on: "Would that include going to Rishikesh, India, for a month-long, 200-hour, yoga/meditation teacher training with my all-time favorite Indian yogi?"

Shaking his head, he answered, "I have a feeling you are not kidding. Please do not be a jackass. Enjoy India!"

That is how I ended up at Swasti Yoga on the banks of Mother Ganga training to be a yoga teacher with my dear guru, Surinder Singh.

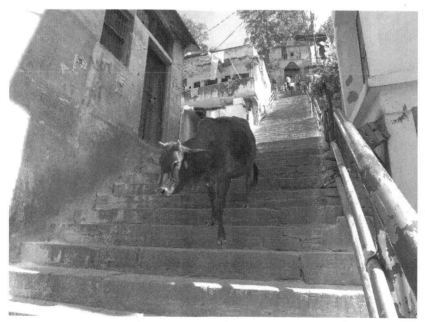

Only in India

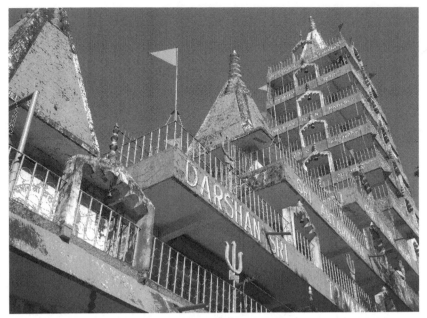

Rishikesh Temple

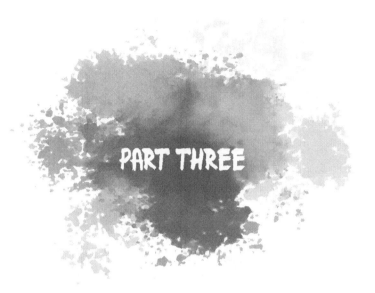

PART THREE

Yoga Teacher Training

During my second trip to India, I sat in Surinder's class one day thinking about his teacher training. Using simple logic, I determined that my mood improved each time I went to his drop-in class. If one hour per day was good, why not sign up for a month-long training?

When Dr. Chopp gave me the green light to travel and practice yoga again, I immediately visited the Swasti Yoga website. Naturally, a teacher-training course was listed that fit ideally with my shoulder recovery. I began making preparations for a third trip to India.

Expectations

When I am preparing to travel, friends often ask me, "Are you excited about your trip? What are you going to do when you get there?" Most of my trips are for at least a month, so these are logical questions that are always asked with good intentions. Unfortunately, such questions totally miss the mark of any journey.

Excitement requires attention to be subtracted from the current moment. It also sets the hook for an attachment to a future event that may or may not happen.

Prior to going to India for my third trip, I knew that I would live in the ashram for 10 days, then move to the yoga shala and take a teacher training that would last a month. I was also hopeful that I would reconnect with friends from my previous visits to the area. I did have one massage booked prior to arrival, but beyond that, I did not set any type of expectations about what would or would not happen.

I would have found it easy to fantasize or daydream about things that might happen. I could have imagined myself meeting my soulmate in the training and falling deeply in love. I could have envisioned a spiritual awakening wherein all my mortal problems would dissipate into space and be replaced with eternal bliss. Given the anticipated level of yoga practice and diet change, it would have been quite logical to imagine some type of transformation in my body. Perhaps six-pack abs?

In each one of these examples, certain expectations could be set. Would my new love be tall? Would I float back home on a magic carpet? Would *AARP Magazine* want to feature me for the "Abs over 50" issue?

Allowing these ridiculous thoughts to gain traction might set a high-water mark that could either be met or not. If not met, would I equate that to failure? If met, would I wonder if I could have done even better?

Yoga teaches a person acceptance. I have learned to enter each practice with the intention of always doing my best to stay in the moment and to achieve stillness in my mind. This intention is extremely different from walking into class with the attitude that today is the day I will hold dancer pose for 90 seconds and my form will be perfect. Again, a ridiculous expectation is established, and judgment comes into play about results that are better or worse than the preconceived notion.

My trips typically begin with flights, which are usually a wonderful place to test acceptance. It is never a clever idea to walk down the jetway with thoughts of being upgraded to first class, of being seated next to fascinating people, of arriving early to a destination. Life is much more interesting when I accept a delayed flight as the universe telling me that I have another purpose in that moment. In my younger days, I would take a delay as a conscious effort on behalf of the CEO of Delta Airlines to purposely ruin my day.

What I do take on every trip now is an intention to be very open to accepting what happens, to letting each day unfold. The best memories of my life always come from the unexpected synchronicities that make each day richer. If coincident events are not happening to me with regularity, the universe is telling me that I am on the wrong path—a cosmic hint to shift gears and change lanes.

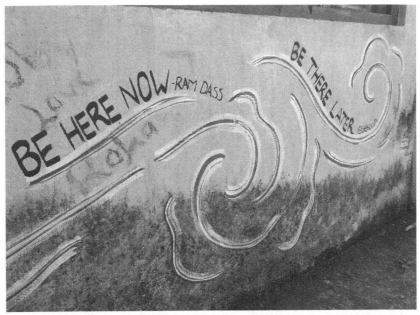

Rishikesh Street Quote

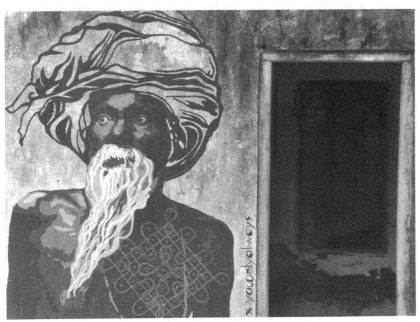

Beatles Ashram Art

Harish Massage Express

Before my 2017 yoga teacher-training course began, I had planned to stay 10 days at Parmarth Ashram. That schedule gave me an opportunity to spend some quality time with my favorite Rishikesh massage therapist, Harish.

I had met Harish the previous year in Rishikesh. During that stay, I had enjoyed many Iyengar yoga classes. This type of yoga focused on alignment and positioning and provided a nice complement to the more traditional classes offered by Surinder. However, when attempting a very unnatural back-bending practice in one class, I felt a movement in my lower back that was not normal. I completed the class but felt some pain after returning to my room. I decided to take a short nap, but when I woke up, I could barely get out of bed.

I sent a few Facebook messages to friends trying to find a local practitioner with chiropractic skills. The first person to respond informed me that there was a spine clinic at the hospital directly behind my ashram. I walked all of two blocks to arrive at the doorstep of this small Indian hospital. A kind young lady asked about my ailment and directed me to fill out a form with three questions. Instead of wanting my payment information, they were interested in my actual problem.

Within minutes, I met with a doctor who did a manual manipulation of my lower spine. The pain dissipated the moment we heard the "click" of something going back to where it belonged. He finished the procedure with ice, electronic muscle stimulation, and therapeutic ultrasound treatment. The doctor recommended a week of rest and as much massage as possible. My hour-long visit cost $4.80.

The doctor's recommendation reminded me of a recent conversation with Kevin, a self-proclaimed massage connoisseur. His enthusiasm for a massage therapist named Harish was so extreme that I added Harish's number to my phone. I never really expected to have a need to call. Well, with my back injury, I was soon grateful for Kevin's advice.

Over a 10-day period, I received seven incredible massages from Harish. My back healed and we began to build a friendship during our sessions.

As I prepared for my third visit to India, I naturally thought again of Harish. I knew my post-surgery shoulder would be in need of a ridiculous amount of loving massage, so I used Facebook messenger to arrange for a two-hour session on my second day in town.

On the scheduled day, I arrived at the Orange Hotel and easily found his new studio below the stairs leading to the lobby. The studio had one desk and two massage rooms with a small mattress on each floor. A few decorations filled the walls, and soothing Indian music set the vibe.

Harish truly had some magic fingers and an intuitive ability to find the tension without being told of its location. I had 10 unencumbered days and ended up on his mats most of those days. When my yoga classes began, I was under more time constraints and told him that our sessions would happen only on rest days (Sundays). He came up with an ingenious idea to eliminate the walking time by providing roundtrip transportation via his scooter. Our meeting place, on the corner of a busy street and a hidden path leading to the yoga shala, was quickly named "the spot" from which the Harish Express facilitated regular massage sessions. The scooter shuttle also amplified his business as my fellow students learned to text him for massage appointments, transportation included.

Toward the end of my trip, Harish expressed an interest in having me share a meal at his home to meet his family. I was honored. We made plans for a massage on a Saturday afternoon to be followed by a late lunch at his home. The day before our meeting, I found out that my yoga group had a rare Saturday afternoon class which would cramp my schedule—I would not have time for both the massage and the lunch. I felt bad and did not know which was more important to him: my meeting his family or his making some income. I deferred the choice to him via a short text message. I was pleased when I read, "It is much more important that you meet my family."

We met at "the spot," and I hopped on the back of his scooter. On my first visit to India, the constant beeping of car horns and meeping from scooters about drove me over the edge. My lifetime experience with honking was from an angry perspective. In the U.S., most people aggressively smashed the middle of the steering wheel, clenched their teeth, and had violent fantasies of running over the person who had somehow violated their space. Worse would be the driver who was not traveling through time at a pace consistent with our own. Probably on purpose. Hooooonkkkkk. In India, the constant meep-meep-beep-beep-meep was so intense that a friend jokingly told me to get a phone app to simulate the sound so my reentry back home would be easier.

On my later trips to India, I was able to view their honking from a new perspective. Most of the large cargo trucks had "BLOW HORN" or "HORN PLEASE" written in foot-high letters on their tailgates. The driver was saying, "I cannot see you, so please give me some noise to feel your presence." The scooter driver was not honking at the pedestrians in anger. Instead, the message was, "I am on your left and do not want to hit your body." What previously seemed to be anger was more like an advanced harmonic communication system built with love.

This new frame of mind allowed me to be a passenger on a scooter and relax into a meditative state. After 15 minutes, we arrived at the end of a winding maze of single-lane streets. Harish tucked the scooter into a walkway leading toward his house.

We walked under a small archway that led to five entrances on each side of the narrow path. Each place was a separate home with shared walls between neighbors. Walking down the path, I asked, "Harish, do you bring clients here often?" I froze when he replied, "You are the first."

Harish's family had lived in this home for 42 years. He had been there for all of his 38 years. He lived there with his mother, father, brother, nephew, wife, son, and daughter. We entered the home and within a few steps were in a cramped kitchen. Six steps away we passed through two wooden doors. Harish said, "This is my room."

A queen-sized bed filled most of the space. Random splotches on the yellow walls of peeling paint exposed the previous turquoise color. A pink floral curtain covered the only small window. Harish and I sat on the bed while his wife, son, and daughter sat 2 feet away on a couch that was three cushions wide. Harish's wife Geeta was dressed in a blue sari over a red traditional dress (Mekhela Sador). Navya, their two-year old daughter, was in a blue and pink onesie, while Omkar, their 10-year old son, wore a bright orange cricket jersey and traditional Western jeans. A cluttered desk stood at the base of the bed. A single 4-foot-wide metal cabinet held the entire wardrobe for this family. The room itself was probably no more than 100 square feet.

Omkar wanted to know which sports I watched, and Geeta was interested in my love life. We took a photo together, and I asked his wife if I could put my arm around her for the picture. Seemingly embarrassed, she said, "I do not think that would be good." On the bed, she then set out two sections of newspaper, which served as placemats for our meal. Harish and I sat cross-legged on the bed and dined on a traditional Indian meal of chapati, dal, cauliflower, and rice pudding. The shared salad was a plate filled with tomato wedges, onions, lime slices, and super-hot green chilies.

As we were enjoying the food, I asked, "Where do the children sleep?"

Harish looked confused and replied, "I do not understand."

I repeated, "Where do they sleep?"

Still bewildered, he answered, "Well, usually my angel Navya is next to me, but sometimes it is Omkar. Why is the order important?"

Humbled, I replied, "You mean we are eating where your entire family sleeps?"

He smiled and said, "Yes, don't spill."

A bit later he mentioned that his mother and father owned another home that had been offered to his family. In that home, they all would have separate rooms. I asked, "Why don't you live there?"

He said, "It is too far and would create too much separation with our family." I asked how far, and he replied, "About a kilometer."

After our lunch, we climbed a few stairs to the roof. Since most homes have no yards and the walls are connected, the flat roofs serve as a social meeting place. Community clotheslines crisscross the roofs and are loaded with the bright colors of drying shirts and pants.

After a lovely afternoon, Harish fired up the "Harish Express" and drove me back to the yoga shala.

At this time, back home in Idaho, I was considering an elaborate remodel of my master bathroom. I was planning a much larger shower, a heated tiled floor, new cabinets, and modern lighting. After my visit to Harish's house, I pulled out my laptop and sent a brief email to my contractor. It read, "Thank you for your bid, but I have decided to pass on this project."

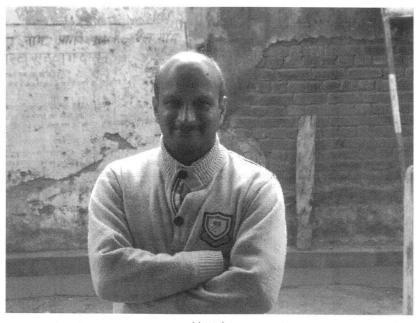

Harish

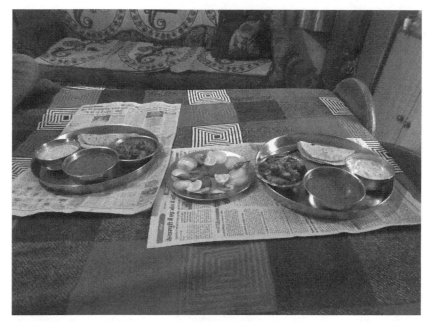

Bed Lunch

Check-In Day

When it was time to move to Surinder's yoga shala for my teacher-training course, Narayan's worker Bablu met me in my room and hoisted my suitcase onto his shoulder. After three years of visiting Rishikesh, I was amazed as he blazed still another alternate path to Surinder's studio. I wondered how many other paths were yet unknown to me.

When we arrived, I realized I had entered these same doors into the lobby at least 40 times over the previous two years, but always as a drop-in student. This time, I was crossing the same threshold to begin a month-long journey with strangers from around the world. The teacher training was set to begin the next day.

The yoga shala building was five stories. The first floor had a reception area, a kitchen, a guest bathroom, and a dining hall. The second, third, and fourth floors each had four guest rooms. The top floor was the yoga studio, with duct tape binding large sheets of thin brown carpet that almost covered a concrete floor. Well-used mats were stuffed into a cupboard next to stacks of fleece blankets. Limp, oblong bolsters were piled high next to various-sized wooden blocks. One final set of stairs led to an open-air rooftop.

To enter my second-floor room, I removed the oversized padlock and slid the black metal bolt to the open position. The modest room had barely enough space for a double bed and a small desk. My closet, 3 feet wide and 4 feet tall, held two hangers. The cramped bathroom was typical with no barrier between toilet and shower. A lone dim light hummed below a noisy bathroom fan. The tiled floor retained a chill from the cooler night's air. Two thick blankets lay folded on top of dull white sheets.

After settling into my new digs, I decided to take an evening stroll to an area called Topovan for some Italian food at VJ's. After a long walk, I was looking forward to some brick-oven margherita pizza. I devoured the food and enjoyed the scenic overview of the river. During the solo meal, my mind consciously wandered into the unknown future with thoughts of the teacher training. Who might I meet? Could I endure the physical aspects? Would my spiritual path broaden?

On the way back to the yoga shala, I ended up on the long set of stairs above the Lakshman Jhula Bridge. The iron suspension structure, built in 1929, spanned 450 feet across the Ganges River. With my eyes and mind on the view, I missed the last step and came crashing down. My right knee already had issues, and my entire body weight was now twisting the joint in a very unnatural manner. I crumbled backward and toward the left. My left forearm took the brunt of the fall as it collided with the cold cement stair. This crash felt like my Costa Rica wave wreck all over again.

Three deep, distinct gashes ran up from my wrist to my elbow. Each cut was aligned with the point of impact from the stair. Adrenaline put me back on my feet, although my knee made an audible noise with each movement. With blood dripping from my wounds, I somehow managed to walk back to the yoga shala.

Surinder's cook, who is also the night watchman, met me at the front door. His eyes told me I looked bad. He pulled out an ancient first-aid kit and began to fumble around for useful items. I made a beeline to the bathroom to wash the wounds with soap and water. My white T-shirt looked like a costume from a horror movie. I used some toilet paper as a compress and returned to the cook.

I was quite sure the first-aid kit had not been replenished as it lacked common items like gauze, antibiotic ointment, and tape. We improvised by covering each cut with small stacks of napkins and then securing them in place with duct tape. Without many other options, I ascended the stairs for my first night at the yoga center.

On the landing, I also met my first classmate, Christian from Ecuador. Using his thumb and forefinger, he stroked his beard while apparently trying to make sense of a 6-foot-5 bald American with blood-soaked napkins, secured by three strips of silver tape, on his arm. Feeling defeated, I entered my room, took six Advils and drifted off to sleep.

I awoke the next morning with throbbing pain in my right knee, which was not a great beginning for the first day of a month-long, 200-hour yoga teacher training. After hobbling to the bathroom, I ripped off the cook's duct tape. The adhesive did a superb job of depilating my arm. After observing my semi-hairless arm under the dim light, I washed off the crusted blood with soap and water in the tiny bathroom sink. I stepped back into the main room and used the natural window light for a better visual inspection. I was happy to see that the cuts were not dripping blood, but my forearm looked like a bad tattoo sleeve done by an angry artist. The cuts were framed by a disgusting bruise in several shades of black, blue, and purple.

Since the training class was not set to begin until 3 p.m., I decided to hobble up the three flights of stairs to see if my abused body was capable of surviving the drop-in class. Except for my injured knee, partially healed shoulder, and kaleidoscope-colored arm, everything was just peachy.

The two-hour class usually flew by, but on this day it seemed like a week. Instead of connecting with my inner bliss and stillness, my mind drifted into dark torture dungeons. I almost cried with happiness when Surinder told us to relax into the closing shavasana pose.

Surinder had no idea of my previous night's injuries, but his words during the resting pose seemed to be tailored to my situation. He spoke about how nature would not always give us what we want, but would always give us what we need. I used these words to exit the self-pity pool and focus on gratitude. My arm was not broken, my knee was functional, and I was about to embark on a life-changing month with strangers from all corners of the world.

On the way out of class, a beautiful young lady asked if I was taking the teacher training. Long locks of wavy hair flowed from under her straw hat. Ani, probably in her mid-20s, became my new German friend. She invited me to lunch, but I had already planned to visit Harish to see if his magic fingers could alleviate some of my knee pain.

After the massage, I returned to my bed for a quick nap. Around 2:30 p.m., I exited my room to begin my teacher training.

I had been in this studio so many times, but nothing was like this experience. The class included 16 students and four teachers. Three men and 12 women were my classmates. We were from Poland, Australia, Italy, Iran, Ukraine, Holland, Spain, Canada, France, Germany, England, USA, and Portugal. At 53, I was 12 years older than the next-oldest, and 30 years older than the youngest. I even had a three-year lead on Surinder. How had I become "the old guy"?

For some reason, I had thought Surinder would lead all the sessions, but that was just not practical. While he was the heart and soul of the training, his brother was there to teach anatomy, a second teacher taught philosophy, and a third was responsible for chanting and meditation. However, Surinder did instruct the bulk of the time, with four hours of asana practice each day.

After brief introductions, Surinder and the teachers opened all the exterior windows and began placing small pieces of wood into a portable square metal fire pit. They poured ghee onto the wood to begin an elaborate ceremony, a combination of puja and havan. This ancient practice was meant to purify the participants and the learning environment.

Swami Atma chanted the mantras as we students took turns sitting by the flames and rhythmically placing offerings into the fire. These offerings included whole grains, marigolds, seeds, rice, nuts, and dried fruit. The ceremony concluded with the tying of red and yellow sacred Hindu threads (Kalava) on our wrists to signify unity.

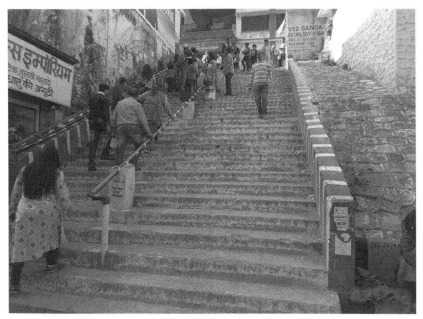

Crash Site

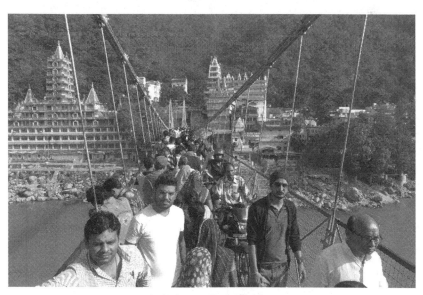

Lakshman Jhula Bridge

Juan and Sona

When I left my room on the first day of training, my timing was in unison with my neighbors across the hall. Our doors opened simultaneously, and that moment was my first encounter with Juan and Sona. Juan introduced himself as "Whooo-Waaaaaan." He turned a single-syllable name into two syllables, with the accent squarely placed on the second. The enunciation lasted an entire exhale cycle. His black wiry hair was held tight to the skull with a man bun. A scraggly beard and mustache contained a few gray hairs that had been earned over the previous 42 years. In a grand manner, he said, "I am from Argentina, and this is my wife, Sona." When his hazel eyes squinted, I could tell there was a very inquisitive nature about this man. With a warm handshake, I said, "Nice to meet you. I am Kurt, and I live in the United States."

Juan was a manly man, and Sona was pure feminine energy. Her softness began with her smooth, wrinkle-free face. Her healthy lifestyle gave her the look of being in her late 20s. I was amazed to learn that my estimate was light by 10 years. Long dark wavy hair, parted in the middle, framed a narrow face with large brown eyes and a warm smile. She spoke slowly and softly and always asked penetrating questions. Sona was born in Iran but was forced to flee the country when she was six. As a couple, they seemed to be tuned into each other's thoughts. One would ask a question, and they would both patiently wait for the answer. Their thirst for spiritual knowledge seemed to be insatiable. They both had fat, leather-bound journals, in which they wrote tiny words on page after page.

They had wandered and wondered the world together. When I asked about their plans after the teacher training, Sona looked at me with a puzzled face and said, "Maybe Thailand or Nepal. We are here now, so there is no reason to worry about what happens next. We prefer what is happening now."

Every day throughout the training, they were the first two into the fifth-floor yoga studio. They always took the front row by Surinder and arrived early for a minimum 30 minutes of meditation.

On the second day of class, Juan pulled his hair out of the man bun and a new person emerged. The monkish meditator with tightly bound hair became a handsome man of the world with a movie-star mane. His boisterous locks perfectly framed his larger-than-life personality.

Throughout the training, I often enjoyed time outside the yoga shala with Juan and Sona. Together we walked along Mother Ganga, visited Lakshman Jhula for meals, or just hung out on the open-air rooftop. We always greeted each other with warm smiles and frequent group hugs.

About two weeks into the program, I was walking by the Ayurvedic Café and saw Sona standing in the doorway. With the light behind her, she looked angelic. I threw my arms around her, and Juan quickly joined the party.

Sona rested her hands on my shoulders and said, "Kurt, we were just talking about you. Each day at dinner, you share upbeat stories about your day. India is very dirty, but by looking at your Facebook photos, you would think we are living in an art gallery. Hugs and smiles are your trademark. I really think that *our* main purpose in this yoga training is to emulate some of the goodness that *you* seem to find around every corner."

I ran into them on my final day in Rishikesh. They had moved out of the yoga shala and into a guesthouse. Since the training was over, they were open to talking about travel destinations. We considered Greece, Turkey, Costa Rica, and Bali. I asked, "What about the United States?"

Juan looked toward the ground and with a sly smile said, "We are not very fond of the U.S. politics."

I said, "That's understandable, but why judge an entire country based on the current leadership? They come and go. In the meantime, we have beautiful national parks and some incredible landscapes. There are some very nice people, too."

Juan laughed and said, "You have a point about judgments. On the first day when we saw your shaved bald head and you said USA, I thought the fucking Marines had landed!" Afterward, I asked Sona, "How are we going to live with this man for a month?"

We shared a final group hug, and Juan took a mala bead bracelet off his wrist and put in on mine. "There are 22 black beads and one silver Buddha face," he said. "We are the silver link, so we will always be with you and watching you."

I said, "What happens when there are things you should not see?"

Sona laughed and replied, "Please twist the bracelet in a manner that will give you some privacy."

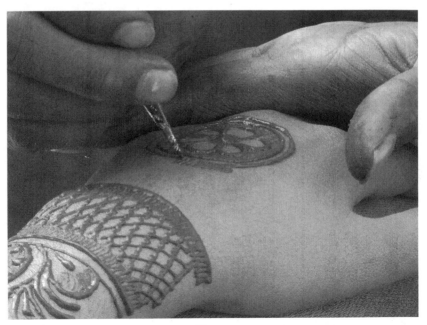

Henna

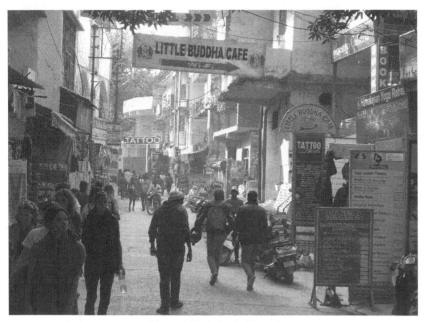

Typical Rishikesh Street

Daily Grind

During our yoga training kick-off ceremony, I asked if there was a daily plan. Surinder smiled and directed us to the schedule posted on the tiny bulletin board on the first floor. The lone item on the corkboard was held in place by four pushpins. The schedule had been copied so many times that it was completely off-center and a faded shade of gray.

The schedule showed no dates because when Surinder did teacher trainings, the schedule did not change. Sunday was completely omitted because it was our day of rest. Monday through Saturday began at 6:30 a.m. for two hours of asana and pranayama. While we enjoyed our group breakfast at 8:30 a.m., Surinder taught the drop-in community practice. For these sessions, we always had the option to participate or observe.

On several occasions, I took advantage of the opportunity to observe the community practice. Since I had taken so many of these classes during past visits to Rishikesh, becoming the observer provided a nice change of perspective. Even when the yoga mats were positioned just inches apart, Surinder floated through the room like a skilled dancer. Using nonverbal communication, he would point to a student and then gesture with his hands to shape a pose, offer a smile to admire a skill, or pull a frown to indicate an improper position.

Surinder used a gentle approach to adjust the yogis. For lengthening, he might touch an outer thigh with his fingernails and scratch outward. For elevating hips in a downward dog, he would lightly place his middle finger on a hip bone and pull up. As the student responded, he was always quick to say, "Thiiiiiiiiiiis is gooooood," followed by an encouraging pat on the back. Often, I would even see him adjust one student using his hands while simultaneously adjusting another participant with his toes.

After breakfast ended at 9:30 a.m., we had self-study time until 11 a.m. Like school kids, we often abused this freedom to sneak into town for lattes and chocolate peanut butter balls. On the days of obedience, I would take my 200-page study guide to the best classroom on the planet—the sandy beach on the banks of Mother Ganga.

From 11 a.m. to 12:30 p.m., we studied yoga anatomy and physiology with Surinder's brother. Gurmeet's teaching style was a bit dry, but the subject of anatomy was rather mechanical by nature. Our classroom was the yoga studio. We sat on the floor or built chairs by stacking bolsters on yoga mats.

A small easel held a dry-erase board for any visuals or notes to be shared by the teacher. Three of the six pens that were used on this board never worked. We all found it rather humorous to watch Gurmeet grab a pen with only a 50% chance of success. A snarl would cross his face when he was on the losing side of the gamble. One day in frustration, he uncapped another pen, and when it did not write either, he opened the fifth-story window and threw it out. He had littered, with absolutely no compunction. The entire class exchanged bewildered looks with a common thought: "Did that just happen?" Gurmeet clearly sensed our displeasure, but still did not understand. With an equally puzzled look, he said, "What is wrong? It did not work."

Lunch was served at 12:30, followed by a rest period. From 2-3:30 p.m., Surinder's teaching partner Vimal shared his mystical insights into the philosophy of yoga. The bulk of his time covered The Yoga Sutras of Patangali. Surinder returned from 3:45-5:15 to share more asana practice and teaching methodology. A group dinner was served from 6-7 p.m. On Monday, Wednesday and Friday, Swami Atma taught chanting and meditation after dinner, which put a perfect cap on the longer days. On Saturday, instruction ended after the yoga philosophy session at 3:30 p.m. The schedule had a box with five smiley faces in this block and said, "Spend your time wisely."

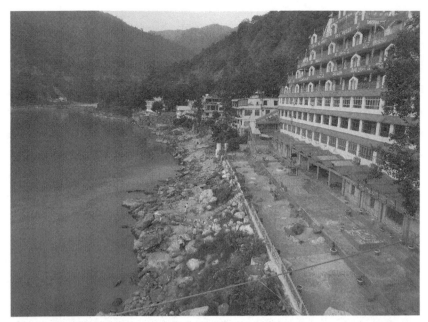

Mother Ganga

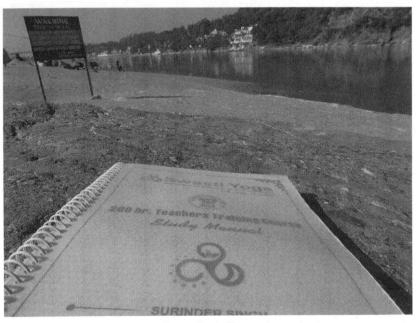

River Study Time

Eva's Sketchnote Book

One day on the yoga mat during my second trip to India, I noticed a mountain of hair piled high in a bun atop a husky man. At the end of the practice, he rearranged his locks into a ponytail that hung well past his midback. After the class wrapped up, he patiently waited for a lady who was busy sketching in an oversized notebook. On the way out of the room, I followed them down the five sets of stairs to the lobby. I introduced myself and was then in the company of Nathanael and Eva.

A few days later, I saw them in one of the endless ATM lines at the State Bank of India during the currency crisis; like I had, they were doing their time in the four-hour line in hopes of getting 20 survival dollars out of the electronic cash dispenser. Noting the copious sweat on Nathanael's forehead, I surmised they were not enjoying their wait.

I stopped by a street vendor and bought some snacks and two bottles of water. Eva and Nathanael were pleased with their gifts, and I had a great excuse to eat a midday samosa. While we ate, I stood in line with them for a bit, which gave us some time to become friends.

The lovely couple from London was on an extended journey around the world. Eva was enrolled in Surinder's teacher training, and Nathanael would join her for the drop-in class afterward. When I asked Eva about her drawings, she explained, "I am a very visual person. It helps me retain the information."

About a week later, I was walking past The Office (another great eatery) and saw the U.K. couple waiting for their food. I ordered a vegetable pancake and some chai and sat with them. I asked Eva if she would share her drawings. With a big smile, she pulled a sketchbook from her backpack and placed it in my hands.

I flipped to a random page and was drawn to a sketch of Surinder's oversized bearded face. He was illustrated in the lotus position with the words "breathe innnnnn" floating above his head. Carefully placed words, large and small, bold and plain, filled out the frame. They read: "The best thing that happened today. The day already started off lovely with a little chai on the way to yoga. Then a fantastic yoga class with Surinder, who is a lovely, calm, gentle person, who gives great subtle correction and oozes calm positivity." She had also sketched the entire class from that day. Each pose was illustrated with a two-inch body and arrows visually explaining where each body part was meant to be and how the muscles should be stretched, contracted, or rotated.

Several months later and back in Boise, I was preparing for my annual trip to Palm Springs with my mom. I was hoping to practice some yoga and thought about buying a book of poses. Instead, I sent a Facebook message to Eva asking if she would be willing to share some of her sketches. My email inbox was soon filled with seven pages of her work. Eva also mentioned that she was making a "sketchnote" book named *Notes from Yoga Teacher Training.*

A year later, the beautiful published book accompanied me into my own yoga teacher training with Surinder.

During a scheduled break several days into the training, I joined three of my yoga classmates for a short walk to Lakshman Jhula for lattes and peanut butter chocolate balls. We found the goods at The Pumpernickel German Bakery. We were lucky to get a table overlooking the Freedom Café and the mighty Mother Ganga. A sign above our table read, "No Smoking Weed Ji." A very polite prohibition, given the "ji," a common term of respect.

We began telling our individual stories of how we chose Surinder's training. Sophie gave a long statement about being super diligent with research by reading blogs, interviewing past participants, and almost ordering a book with drawings from a previous student.

I laughed and asked, "Oh, you mean Eva's book?"

"Get out," she answered. "This cannot be. Are you sure it's the same author?"

"Not only am I sure, but she will be here in a week," I confirmed. "Would you like me to have her bring a book for you?"

I did a quick Google search on my phone and suspended Sophie's disbelief by showing her an image of the book cover. Eva was pleased to hear from me and agreed to bring a few copies for her upcoming trip to Rishikesh.

Several weeks later, while on a walkabout, I was enjoying refreshments at The Juice House when Eva and Nathanael, who had recently returned to Rishikesh, passed on the street. They joined me on a bench, Eva on my right and Nathanael on my left. When Vishvas arrived for his daily shift of juice-making, I introduced him to my friends. Although he was anxious to get to work, he quickly said, "Kurt, I have a favor to ask of you. Some of your fellow students were here yesterday, and they had a little book with drawings of yoga poses." I glanced at Eva and reveled in her beaming grin. He continued, "Do you think you could find a way for me to buy that book?"

"Well," I said, "I know the author. She sold her last book to one of my yoga classmates earlier today, but I bet you could make arrangements to get one from her."

Much to his surprise, Eva piped in then and said, "I have one copy left, and it's the one I use to show people my work. But, I feel that it needs to be yours, so I will bring it for you tomorrow."

Visibly moved, Vishvas responded, "Oh what a great honor." Then he asked, "How much would that cost me?"

Eva looked toward the sky, squinting her eyes in thought before replying, "One juice would be a good trade. The price is one juice."

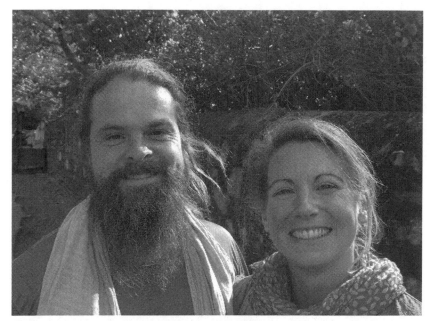

Eva and Nathanael

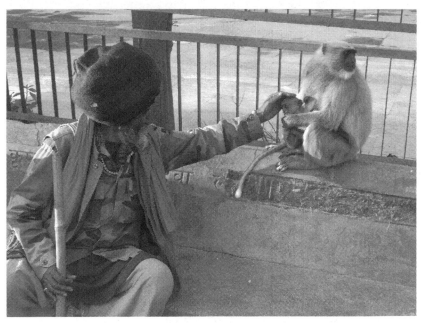

Sharing the Love

On the Road with Arpit

Arpit's father owns a local Rishikesh restaurant that serves traditional Indian dishes along with a wide variety of cuisines including Chinese, Israeli, Italian, and American. I still laugh at the idea of ordering thali, margherita pizza, fries, and vegetable chow mein from the same menu. Arpit manned the cashier station and was always friendly and inquisitive during our exchanges. At the end of my second trip to India, we became Facebook friends. Over the next year, we exchanged a few messages to keep in touch.

On my third trip, he was quite happy to see me and asked if we could spend some time together. We made plans to meet the following night at 8 p.m. I assumed that we would get a quick cup of java. Well, after eating a big meal, I met at the assigned time and was looking forward to some coffee and dessert at the nearby café. Upon arrival he smiled and said, "Hop on my bike. I am so hungry. We are going for pizza." Moments later we were weaving in and out of traffic for a few miles on the way to Topovan.

We arrived at VJ's Italian restaurant. The open-air dining area had a few covered tables, but the gems were on the grassy hilltop with panoramic views of Rishikesh. The mighty Ganges looked a bit tamer from this elevated distance. Arpit took charge and ordered pizza, spaghetti, and a sandwich.

Arpit then began sharing his plans for life—plans as big as his appetite. At the ripe age of 20, the only thing holding him back was his intense loyalty to family.

I asked him why he had so much interest in dining with me. "You are twice my age and have seen things I will never see," he said. "I would like to learn from you." I tried to put myself in his shoes at that age and could not imagine myself seeking anything other than self-gratification.

During our dinner, we made plans to visit Devprayag, the sacred confluence where the Alaknanda and Bhagirathi rivers merge to forge the headwaters of Mother Ganga. Although Devprayag is located just 40 miles from Rishikesh, the trip takes at least two hours in a cab and is ill-advised to attempt without Dramamine. Arpit asked, "Mr. Kurt, would you mind if I brought my girlfriend on this trip?" I replied that I would look forward to meeting her.

A few days later, we met at the taxi stand behind Parmarth where a Tata was waiting to take us upstream. The car arrived at 8 a.m. and was reserved until 5 p.m. for a total cost of $30. Arpit, lugging a small blue backpack, arrived alone. "Is your girlfriend coming?" I inquired.

He said, "It is a problem you will likely not understand. For an Indian girl to take this kind of journey, she would need permission from her parents. She was afraid to tell them about you and was considering leaving that part out. I took back the invitation, so she would not be tempted to dishonor her parents with a story that did not match reality." I tried to compare my modus operandi at his age and silently shook my head in awe of his character.

I asked, "How many times have you been to Dev?"

He shocked me by replying, "Never."

After the stomach-churning drive, we stepped out of the car for our first view of the merging rivers. The Bhagirathi begins at the foot of the Gangotri Glacier. The glacial meltwater, cloudy with minerals, arrives at the confluence violently, as rapids. The Alaknanda begins at the Indian border with Tibet. This glassy river is a deep shade of teal. While smooth and graceful, the Alaknanda's powerful flow has carved an ancient path into the solid rock canyon walls.

The merging occurs at a large ghat stairway built into the natural rock. From above and for about a quarter of a mile, there appears to be a distinct squiggly line as the gray and teal waters unite and eventually become a single body with gorgeous turquoise hues.

We descended about 50 stairs to the yellow suspension bridge that crossed the raging Bhagirathi. The bridge, built for scooter and foot traffic, was obstructed by a lone cow sprawled out, lounging. Like us, she was just enjoying the view.

After a quick chai break, we climbed more than 100 stairs to arrive at the Raghunathji Temple. This temple, established in the eighth century, had a cubed, chimney-like structure that towered above a myriad of pastel-colored homes. We were lucky to arrive just in time for a Hindu service that began with the ringing of the 15 large bells hanging from long chains.

To arrive at the actual river ghat, we descended another 50 to 60 stairs. I stripped down to my underwear, stabilized myself with one of the long chains provided for safety, and stood knee deep in the cool waters. For a small fee, a local Hindu filled my hands with marigolds and water while chanting a prayer for me. An uplifting spiritual energy flowed at this divine location.

We crossed another suspension bridge above the calmer river. Arpit bought a bag of peanuts from a local vendor and shared them with me, a cow, and a kitten.

After several hours of wandering, we reversed course and walked back to the taxi. After driving about half a mile, Arpit asked the driver to pull over.

"Why are we stopping?" I asked.

"We cannot make such a long journey home without a proper lunch," Arpit answered.

"But we do not have any food," I observed. "What are we going to eat?"

Arpit unzipped the blue backpack and spread a sheet of newspaper on the backseat of the car. He then pulled out several containers covered in foil. With a big smile, he said "My mom has prepared our afternoon meal. She told me to tell you hello and to enjoy the offering."

We devoured Mama's chana masala (chickpea dish), tomatoes, cucumber, hot chilis, and paratha (flatbread). With full bellies and enlightened hearts, we began the two-hour drive back home to Rishikesh.

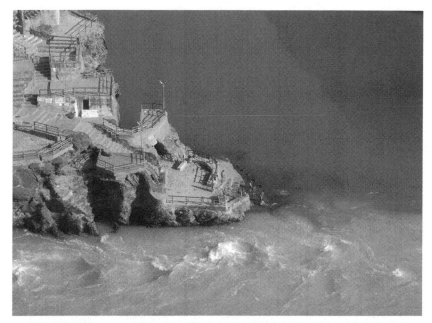

Devprayag

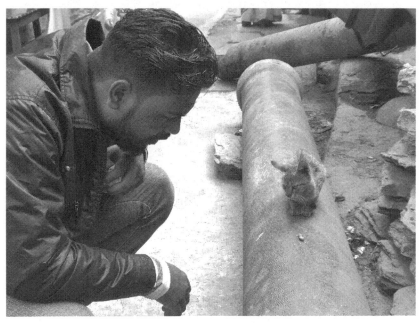

Always Sharing

Twisted

Meals with Harish and Arpit reminded me of lessons I was studying in the anatomy and physiology portion of my teacher training.

Twisting is a regular feature of any yoga practice, and I had learned multiple twisting poses. For example, one involved sitting upright in a chair with my feet facing forward and firmly planted on the ground. Without moving hips or feet, I rotated my shoulders ninety degrees (or as far as possible without strain). The benefits of this pose are widely recognized and include reducing stress, improving flexibility, reduction in lower back pain, and improved digestive function.

In a twisted position, the digestive organs are compressed and temporarily experience constricted blood flow. When the pose is released, fresh blood rushes to the area, delivering new supplies of oxygen and nutrients. The effect is like an internal massage for your organs that increases their ability to function.

We are lucky to have such a brilliant system inside our bodies. On a daily basis, we decide what food goes into our mouths. The digestive system prefers kale and quinoa but will also tolerate bad decisions like pepperoni pizza and chocolate eclairs. Our work ends with the lifestyle choices, and then the body takes over. It decides what nutrients to keep and what to flush.

I had also been meditating on using a similar system to process the thoughts that entered and procreated inside my mind. Unlike the digestive system, I had more control over this process.

I started with the input. I could think blueberries, salmon, and avocados, or I could feed my mind fatty, greasy thoughts. Unhealthy thoughts would always register a negative emotion, like fear or anger. Like attracted like, so I tried to populate my mind with positive thoughts.

Many people might say, "You are what you eat." I would expand that to, "You become what you think."

Since my yoga training, I have become more proactive with my thoughts. I strive to mine the good nutrients from the positive thoughts and use them as a source of energy. When I detect negative thoughts and emotions, I avoid blocking or stuffing them. Undigested foods kill the body just as undigested thoughts pollute the mind. Instead I do my best to feel the negative thoughts, then process and release them.

A short poem by Frank Outlaw sums this idea up for me:

Watch your thoughts, they become words.
Watch your words, they become actions.
Watch your actions, they become habits.
Watch your habits, they become your character.
Watch your character, it becomes your destiny.

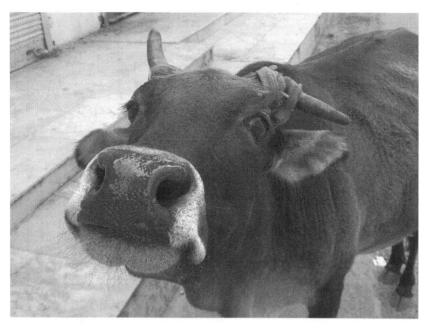

Feed Me

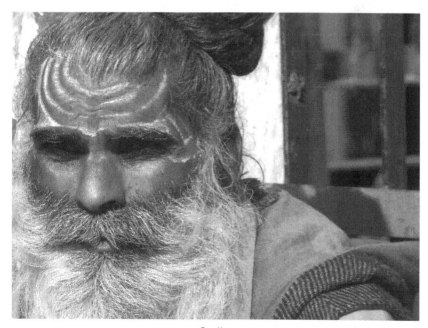

Sadhu

Toxic Gossip

Negative words can be as dangerous and harmful as negative thoughts. This lesson was brought home to me during my yoga training as well, although the instruction had begun three years earlier on a trip to another country with a long tradition of spiritual development.

That journey began in May of 2014 when I was invited to speak to a local book club about my Camino book, *A Million Steps*. Prior to that event, I had met the hostess but knew little more than her name. She lived on Idaho's Payette River in a remote spot about 50 miles from my home. The drive was refreshing as it took me out of the city and back into nature. At least 20 miles of the trip followed the river, which was raging with fresh melting snowpack.

Her book group included about 20 people. One of the first guests to arrive was a local man who told me that he built custom furniture with local materials. My heart skipped a beat when he told me that among his favorite products were his large chairs made from bent willows. About 15 years earlier, I had purchased two of his chairs at a local art show.

As the night was winding down and people were pitching in to clean up, the hostess approached me and said, "This may sound weird, but I am going to Bhutan with four local friends in October. We are doing a cultural tour. After the tour, they depart and I am staying for a 17-day guided hike through the Himalayas. There is room for you."

I had never heard of Bhutan but asked her to send me an email with the details. By the time I arrived home, an email had arrived.

I did some research to investigate further. With Google Maps I found the small landlocked country surrounded by China, Nepal, and India. I learned that two-thirds of the 750,000 residents were Buddhists and the other third practiced Hinduism. Realizing that their country could never compete with larger nations on an economic basis, the Bhutanese advertised that they were the country of "Gross National Happiness." I was immediately hooked and signed up for the three-week trip in October, with 17 of those days dedicated to the Chomolhari-Laya Gasa Trek.

Five months later, our international group of strangers united at the Paro Airport in the capital of Bhutan. We came from Canada, the United States, Singapore, Holland, Hong Kong, Switzerland, and Australia. Notable among us was a married couple from Canada, whose wife's attendance was secured with the bribe of a new home for completing the walk. From the first step, she made it apparent that her reasons for being there began and ended with the new home.

I remember waking on the first day in a tent by the side of a river. Steam fog was pouring off the river and the sun was breaching the horizon. While walking across a field, I ran into the bribed wife on the way to the breakfast table. I tried to share my euphoria but was greeted with complaints about the temperature and the noise from barking dogs. She had a rather gloomy outlook for the day's hike.

Her pessimism did not bode well for the trip because we were effectively tied together for the entire 17-day trek. All meals were shared, and our tents were placed side by side. During the day, we did have a chance to spread out on the trail, but we always stayed within about five minutes of each other.

In my younger days, I would have been a fountain of gossip about this woman, seizing all opportunities to complain about her. She was quite obviously grating on everyone, and not just me. I could have easily started a conversation by saying, "Did you hear…?"

It took me 50 years to reach this point, but instead of stoking a hot fire, I poured cool water on the flames. I took a small leap of faith and decided that she did not wake up every day with the intention to make my day miserable. In her presence, I practiced compassion. When I was not in her presence, I did not allow her to rent any space in my mind.

This experience in Bhutan came to mind on the third week of my yoga training, on a day when I enjoyed lunch conversation with my 29-year-old French friend, Mylena. The previous day, our entire group had traveled with Surinder to watch the sunrise at the Kunjapuri Temple. After only a 30-minute drive, we were gifted with some incredible views of the snow-capped Himalayas.

During the lunch, Mylena made a comment about how the trip helped to calm some tension within our group. I was oblivious to the drama and asked, "What are you talking about? I do not see any drama. What happened?"

She replied, "Why breathe life into a situation that is best left to die?"

I briefly flashed back to Bhutan and remembered my experiences on that walk. I smiled and thought about how lucky Mylena was to learn this lesson at such a young age.

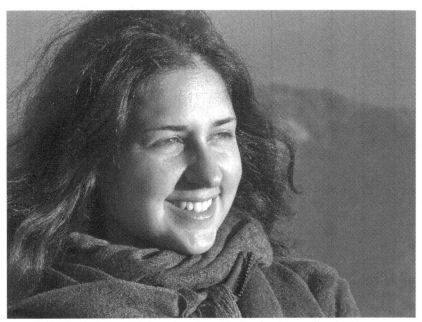

Mylena

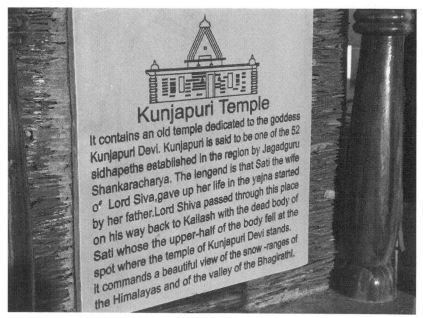

Kunjapuri Temple

It contains an old temple dedicated to the goddess Kunjapuri Devi. Kunjapuri is said to be one of the 52 sidhapeths established in the region by Jagadguru Shankaracharya. The lengend is that Sati the wife of Lord Siva,gave up her life in the yajna started by her father.Lord Shiva passed through this place on his way back to Kailash with the dead body of Sati whose the upper-half of the body fell at the spot where the temple of Kunjapuri Devi stands. it commands a beautiful view of the snow -ranges of the Himalayas and of the valley of the Bhagirathi,

Kunjapuri

Tea with Inessa

At first, Inessa appeared in our yoga teacher training class as a quiet and almost mysterious lady from Ukraine. In most types of our spiritual practice, the teachers recommended that we stay detached as an observer, allowing our thoughts to float in and out of our minds like clouds passing in the sky. Inessa seemed to be a chronic observer of all things. A bit hidden in a shadow, but completely attuned.

Her narrow face was surrounded by wiry, jet-black hair. The shoulder-length locks were a bit disheveled but in a manner that fashion models paid top-dollar to emulate. Her piercing eyes were gray with a hint of blue. I would have guessed her age to be around 35.

A few days into the training we found ourselves sitting together at the breakfast table. I had a small jar of peanut butter that I used to liven up the bland oatmeal. I cracked through Inessa's first shell by offering a dollop for her porridge. She responded with a beautiful, warm smile.

Inessa reminded me of Matryoshka nesting dolls. Each layer that she opened exposed a surprising dimension of her bright soul. When I told her of my plans to visit Devprayag, the headwaters of the Ganges River, she requested that I bring her a liter of water from that sacred spot. Mother Ganga's water had long been thought to have healing abilities. It cleansed the outer body and bathed the soul.

One morning, Inessa invited a group of yoga students for tea and meditation on the ghat. I envisioned us stopping at a tea stall, buying some chai, and relaxing by the water. She asked me to select one of my favorite spots for the outing. I felt like the Pied Piper walking down Sadhu Samajh

138

Market Road followed by Inessa, Juan, Maria, Sona, and Christian. I led them to one of my favorite ghats downstream from the Parmarth Ashram. When we arrived, I said, "We forgot to get tea!"

Inessa slyly grinned and said, "We have all we need … and more."

We sat in a circle on a small concrete ledge about 3 feet from the waters of the Ganges. The flowing water drowned out all the surrounding chaos and noise. Inessa unzipped her small backpack.

She carefully placed a brown towel on the water-worn concrete. In the center of the towel, she set a bamboo tea tray. The tray held a purple teapot, three white teacups, three light teal teacups, and one clear glass pitcher. Inessa had preheated the sacred water from Devprayag and carried it in a well-used metal thermos.

The more formal ceremony began when she took a pinch of black leaves from the first of three tea sachets and placed the loose leaves in a gray porcelain crucible speckled with black dots. Using both thumbs and both forefingers, she gently handed the filled container to Juan and asked that we smell and observe the raw leaves with our hearts only, to leave the mind out of the process. The leaves slowly made their way around the circle. We did this with three different types of tea and ultimately selected one using group heart consensus. Like yoga, this ceremony was a process of union. A connection.

She began the process of making the tea by adding leaves to the strainer, pouring heated water from the small glass pitcher through the leaves, placing the lid on the small purple pot, and then gently swishing the water. The finished tea was returned to the glass pitcher and then distributed into the tiny tea cups sitting on the bamboo tray. Each cup was filled with one sip of tea. One at a time, we were told to take our cup and drink the tea.

After the first round, she said, "The tea was created mindfully by this group. The water mixed with the leaves in an alchemy-like process in the one pot. I again created separation by pouring the tea into individual cups. By allowing the tea into our bodies, we are removing separation and becoming one."

For the next round, she said, "Pay attention to where the tea goes after it enters your mouth."

I internally rolled my eyes and was quite skeptical, but on my next sip, I felt the tea enter my mouth and glide down the back of my esophagus. At my sternum it took a left turn and went directly to my heart. The third round and every subsequent sip took the exact same path. I glanced at Sona and asked, "Where did your tea go?"

Without hesitation she replied, "Directly to my mind."

Inessa explained, "Tea has its character, but it can express itself in your space. All of the spaces inside of us are different, and that is a reason we have different feelings."

We continued this process for a total 12 rounds of tea. The only reason we quit was due to a pending class. On the way back to the yoga shala, I asked Inessa, "How many times have you done that ceremony?"

She replied, "Since 1999, I do it for people every day. I accept it as my lifestyle."

I was honored to see another layer of the nesting doll.

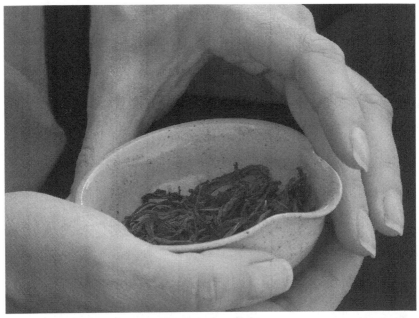

Tea Selection Time

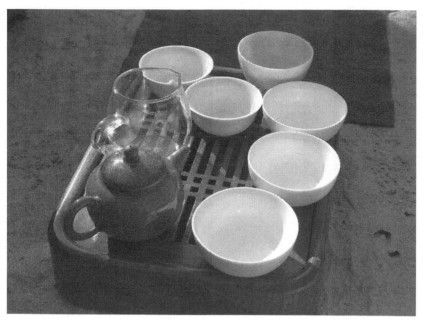

Tea Set

Cremation on the Ganges

On a random day I was wandering around the grounds of Parmarth and visiting with friends. When the river was in view, I noticed a small gathering of people in the process of creating a pyre for a cremation across the water. My intuition told me this was the time for me to observe this ceremony.

I had to walk a half-mile upstream, across the Ram Jhula Bridge, and a bit more than a half-mile down the other bank. While crossing the bridge, I saw a large plume of dense smoke arising from my destination. I felt some immediate relief that I would not actually see the corpse burn. With solemn determination, I walked along the ghat steps leading toward the flames.

Realizing this ceremony was a sacred moment for the friends and family, I made a conscious decision to keep my distance. I sat on a rock, placed my hands at my chest, palms pressed together in the namaskar mudra position, and began the observation.

Throughout our yoga teacher training, Surinder regularly reminded us that we are all made from the five basic elements of earth, water, fire, air, and space. Earth is not just dirt but includes every natural solid like bones, flesh, and hair. With a lower density, water is the base of blood, saliva, semen, and urine. Fire enables the body to digest food and ignite the mind to digest thoughts. Air is less dense than water and permits expansion and contraction within the body. Space exists as mouth, abdomen, ears, nostrils, allowing for vibrations that lead to connection and sound.

From where I sat observing the funeral pyre, I looked out on sand and melon-shaped boulders, the smallest being grapefruit-sized and the larger ones about the size of the iconic Volkswagen Bug. This dense foundation was earth.

Mother Ganga was water and, for me, a real-life manifestation of divine feminine energy. At this spot, the water was smooth yet swirling in many directions at one time, almost as if dancing before my eyes. The softness of the surface of the Ganges disguised the intense power of the river below as she flowed at almost half a million cubic feet per second.

At the cremation pyre, the actual flame appeared as the third tier above the earth and water. The fire would burn for about six hours and consume almost 1,000 pounds of wood. As the flames raged toward the sky, the dense smoke was replaced with clear visible waves as the hot air intersected with the cooler air. Above everything, I was gazing at the forested Himalayas and the blue sky that extended into infinite space.

I sat on my rock in a deep state of personal reflection with my hands pressed together above my heart and elbows pointing toward the ground. My eyes opened and closed while all five elements mixed in front of me. I observed my teachings until one of the men near the fire began to walk toward me.

The man, in his mid-40s, kindly looked into my eyes and asked, "What do you think of this?"

I responded, "In my country, when someone dies, we call the coroner and the body is quickly removed from the premises. If cremation is selected, it is done in seclusion by strangers in a sterile environment. If burial is selected, then we fill the body with chemicals and paint unnatural faces with makeup."

He said, "That does not sound like an effective way to release the soul. If not done properly, the soul will not find a path into the afterlife. We use fire to purify and to scare away harmful demons and spirits."

I noticed that several of the participants were now walking up the river bank about 10 yards and then walking back to the flames. Each person took a handful of water and splashed some on their own face, then took a second handful and added to the fire. I asked, "What are they doing?"

He replied, "They are symbolically aiding the body into Mother Ganga."

"May I participate?" I asked.

He said, "I am not sure but will find out." He approached the larger group, and now everyone was staring directly at me. One by one, their hands waved me down to the shore where I became a participant in this holy ceremony. I cupped water from Mother Ganga to splash on my face, then on the fire. The water sizzled and was quickly transformed into steam when it met the flames.

We went back to the rock and continued our conversation. I asked, "What is your affiliation to the deceased?"

He said, "That is my grandfather."

I replied, "I am sorry for your loss. Do you and your family live in Rishikesh?"

He said, "No, I am one of 80,000 policemen in Delhi. I drove over yesterday for this service. Would you mind if I took a few selfies of us together?"

In a slight state of shock, I nodded approval, and he extended his arm to start snapping shots.

Shortly after the photo shoot, people began to leave the riverside service. I am not sure why it took me so long to notice, but I was quite disturbed that there had not been a single woman present during this process. I asked why and he responded, "They are not allowed." It was not the time or place to explore the reasons, so I saved this question for Surinder.

I took about 30 minutes to walk back to the yoga shala. Numbed into a serene state of peace, my mind could easily have been on another planet. I soon found Surinder and his eyes became alarmingly large when I said, "Surinderji, I just went to a cremation and I have a few questions." Realizing his sense of panic, I explained that I had both observed and participated with absolute reverence. Surinder's eyes returned to a natural size and the master of breathing resumed a normal breathing pattern.

I asked, "Why are women not allowed at the cremation site?"

He seemed to know this rule would be difficult for me to understand. I tried to imagine myself in a headstand position with a mind wide open to consider his explanation from a different perspective.

He said, "In our culture, we believe that men are born without an innate source of love. Without love, the lack of feeling creates a heavy reliance on logic and reason. The man knows that the body must be purified by fire for the soul to be released. That is why your new friend was engaging in some trivial conversation about his job and took selfies with you. But … selfies? Really?"

I replied, "Yes, it happened. But this reasoning still does not explain why women are seemingly discriminated against in this setting. Can you help me understand?"

He replied, "Since women are pure love and the source of love, they have intense feelings and attachment. If the women became strong enough to watch a loved one burn, then their capacity to love would be diminished. Without love, they would not continue to have children, as having a child is the ultimate act of unconditional love. There is also the possibility that the women's attachment would prevent the soul from being released. I am not asking you to agree, but this is our perspective."

I still had difficulty with this explanation but did find some relief when he further explained that the women were very involved with all aspects of the service. If the deceased was a male, the men prepared the body. The women prepared the deceased female body. The women participated in all aspects, including the walk to the cremation site. One hundred meters from the pyre, the women returned home, and the men completed the process.

At the end of the service, the men walked away from the fire and toward their homes. Two eyes on the front of the head were meant to look forward. The final act of the ritual was to grab a random piece of wood to snap between the fingers and toss over the shoulder. This represented the act of breaking the bond and moving forward.

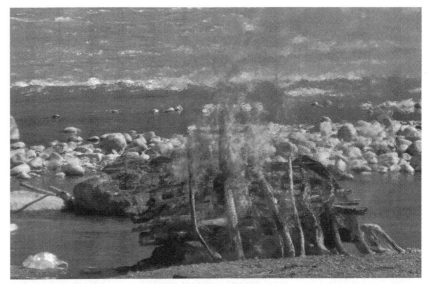

Cremation Pyre

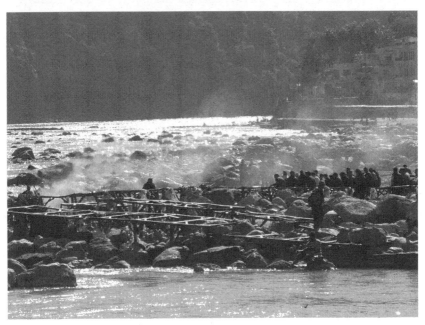

The Service

Deaths in My Family

My experiences with death in India were, in every way, worlds away from the deaths of my grandmother, father, and step-father at home in the U.S.

Grandma Pearl

I was very close to my Grandma Pearl on my father's side of the family. I came into this world on the exact day her husband passed from it. Later in life, I learned that Grampa Ira died from liver failure associated with a life of alcoholism.

In my family, I am the youngest of the three children. Given my mystical bond with my grandma, my parents would often send me to her home for some much-needed rest for themselves.

She was quite poor and lived in a modest home. Somehow, she always found a way to take me to the zoo and for boat rides in the local park. She bought me a seemingly endless supply of peppermint ice cream.

When I was eight years old, her hip problems required some type of surgery, and she went to Oregon for rehabilitation. During that time, I looked forward to the weekly long-distance phone call to hear her voice.

One day, I came home from school, and my brother was adamant that we play a game of ping-pong. He seemed jittery and a bit out of his element on that day. After a few rallies, he paused the game and blurted, "Grandma Pearl is dead."

This shock was my first real-life experience with human death. I was unsure of what it meant to be dead. I asked my brother, "Does that mean she is not coming back home?"

The funeral service ruined me. As a family, we had a front-row seat to an open-casket service. When I had to actually walk up to the casket and view her, I broke into uncontrollable tears. The image of her lifeless, waxy, embalmed face was too much for me. The memory still disturbs me. To this day, I avoid driving by that funeral home.

Dad

In 2001, the call came from my brother. Our dad had been admitted to St. Luke's Hospital in Boise. The same hospital where I was born. The doctors were rather frank that his outlook was not good.

As we waited for the end, I reviewed many fond memories of my father. People gravitated toward his charismatic persona. He had a way of making people feel at ease. He was as equally at home with U.S. Senators in Washington, D.C. as he was with corn farmers in Idaho.

Unfortunately, Dad had little interest in us as children. His main focal points were his legal career and vodka, the emphasis on the latter. As a teenager, I too became fond of drinking beer. I had no idea then such a dangerous fuse had been lit.

Being with Dad was always fun because it meant seemingly endless money, little discipline, and lots of alcohol. In my late teens and early 20s, I watched many people come and go. Wives and law partners were left as road kill. Not me. I was special.

In my mid-20s, I realized he had a big problem with drinking. His problem was so obvious, while I was oblivious to my own. Looking in the rear-view mirror, I did have a father, but our relationship was heavily weighted toward being drinking buddies. By my early 30s, I too became road kill and was replaced with his fourth wife.

When he was at the top of his game, he was one of the sharpest attorneys in the entire Northwest. Despite his alcoholism, one partner once said, "Your dad is better drunk in court than 99% of law grads." A strange, yet honest compliment.

His family and friends tried many times to help him address his addiction problems. I participated in four interventions and bet he had a few more when I was not present. He went to rehab each time and then cheated on his first day out.

Two nights before he died, I sat in his room and stared at my father-friend. His skin was a faded yellow, his mind was gone, and his body bore no signs of his life as a tall, strong man. He was an old, dying man.

By this time, I was well into my own alcoholic lifestyle and had complemented my poor lifestyle choice with an addiction to cigarettes. Sitting by his bedside, I made a commitment to the universe that I would not leave the planet in an analogous manner. I stopped drinking and smoking on that day. As of the writing of this book in 2018, I have been sober and smokeless for 17 years.

Two days later, at the end of my father's life, I chose not to be present due to the scars from my grandmother's passing. I did not want the final image of his off-color, lifeless body. I did not want to know the smell of death.

Stan

My stepfather, Stan, defied all odds in his life. Like my father and me, he began a life of heavy drinking and smoking at a young age. My mother married him when I was 8 years old. For the next 45 years, he drank Scotch whisky to excess and smoked two packs of cigarettes each and every day.

His quality of life was not so good, but his longevity was remarkable. In August of 2017, when Stan was 87 years old, my mom called and said, "I think he is dead. You need to come over now."

I had no question when I arrived. He had passed in his sleep and appeared to be at peace. Unlike my previous experiences with death, this one seemed appropriate. I spent about 10 minutes at his bedside and relived the memories we had shared for a lifetime. I touched his forehead and kissed his cheek, then left the room to call his son, Mike.

Evidently, I was unable to share the news gently. With no preface, I stated: "Stan is dead."

Mike drove to the house. After spending his own time to say goodbye, he joined me and my mom in the kitchen. Being the pragmatic type, he called the funeral home to start the process.

I overheard him say, "No, we have not called 911. Yes, we are sure. Because his lungs are not moving and his body is cooling. OK, I will call them."

He called 911 and explained the situation. I again heard him say, "No, there is no need for EMS. He is deceased. OK. Thank you for not sending them."

Moments later, I heard sirens blazing and saw a bulky red fire truck trying to maneuver down my mother's lengthy driveway. A white ambulance followed. Soon, there were four strangers in the house to confirm Stan was truly dead in his bed. They were all polite, but this procedure seemed a bit much.

The ambulance team left, but the fireman stayed behind. I said, "What is the process, and when do you leave?"

The fireman replied, "When the police get here."

Soon, two squad cars were in the driveway, and three policemen were on the doorstep. The blue team relieved the red team. They were kind and thoughtful and asked some basic questions. I had one of my own: "As a taxpayer, this seems a bit insane. Why are there three of you?" I found a morsel of comfort when one of the policemen said they always send two, but the third man was in training.

As kind as they were, their welcome was beginning to wear thin. Again I asked, "What is the process, and when do you leave?"

The same policeman said, "There is no foul play, but we need the city inspector to come before we can leave."

About 30 minutes later, a brand new white truck with flashing orange lights joined the caravan of vehicles in the driveway. A serious lady stepped out of the car, put on some surgical gloves, and approached the door. Without offering a word of condolence, she said, "Please move to the side. I need room for a clear photo of the entryway and the steps leading to the bedroom. Do not disturb me. I will also need all of his prescription pills." With that breath of fresh air, she snapped her way into the bedroom.

The city inspector was followed by the coroner, who confirmed the death and asked, "Would you like me to call the funeral home?"

By this time, all three of us burst into laughter. My stepbrother said, "Yes. That is what we tried to do four hours ago."

The inspector called but frowned as he hung up the phone. "They are very busy and will try to be here in about 90 minutes," he explained.

Two professional death salesmen later showed up at the door in their finest suits. They had brochures in hand and a gurney. Moments later, Stan was wheeled out of his house in a red velvet body bag. The fancy salesmen left mud stains on the carpet.

That red velvet bag was, for me, the visual symbol of how Americans hide from the death that is exposed in full view on the banks of Mother Ganga. In India, old people are cared for and honored. Death is a natural part of existence. In the West, we see death as unnatural or surreal. We fear, repel, and reject it. In Rishikesh, my accumulated fear of death began to dissolve.

Jeanie's Life Celebration

Not long after I returned from my third trip to India, a close family friend died. The mourning process, this time, provided a completely different experience of death in the U.S. for me. Although sorrowful, the service was also celebratory.

For the previous 27 years, Jeanie had arrived at my home every other Tuesday at 7:45 a.m. to clean my house. Her daughter Janet used to do housekeeping for my father, so these two ladies had been in my life for over 40 years. They were family.

When I heard the rattle of the garage door opening, that was my signal to get a fresh cup of coffee and take it into my home office for some time to catch up with Jeanie. She would drop her supplies in the kitchen and join me. After a hug, she would take her seat on my grandfather's iconic cushioned chair. We would swap stories for 30-45 minutes before she began her work.

I do not think there was another person on the planet who knew more about me than Jeanie did. And this exchange was a two-way street, as I knew her deepest secrets in return. I knew about all her loves and fears, her kids and grandkids, her neighbors and friends. I could tell her mood and health with a glance at her face. When one of us had good or bad news, we supplemented the bi-monthly chats with phone calls to share the freshest tales.

Five years prior to her death, she was diagnosed with an aneurysm near her kidney, a problem usually fixed with a simple surgical procedure. However, due to the location, her surgery would have been very high risk—one she was not willing to endure. For six months after her diagnosis, our Tuesday chats began and ended with tears. Around the seventh month, her more familiar ornery self showed up and declared, "I am not going to let this ruin my life. I now refer to my problem as 'Junior' and will be damned if he will ever drive this train."

As I was writing this book, she called and asked about changing the upcoming regularly scheduled Tuesday to a Thursday due to a paving project around her house. She was concerned about not having access to her car. Of course I agreed, but was personally bummed because I had a two-day trip planned and would miss updating her with the details and photos from my most recent Costa Rica adventure.

When I walked into my house on that Friday at noon, my heart skipped a beat. My house had not been cleaned. For the first time in 27 years, Jeanie no-showed without a call. In panic mode, I dialed her number and left a message. I unsuccessfully tried to call her daughter Janet at about 2 p.m. At 4:00 I once again tried to call Jeanie at home. Around 5:00 she called and said, "I am so sorry. I simply forgot to call. The paving is a nightmare." She then started to ramble about the hassle.

I interrupted her to say, "Jeanie, I know it is a problem, but for the past five hours, I truly thought 'Junior' may have blown and that you were gone. I want you to know in this moment and every other moment how much I love you and appreciate your friendship."

She thanked me but quickly resumed telling me about the paving nightmare. We were both looking forward to catching up on our next scheduled cleaning date.

Five days later, her daughter found her dead of a heart attack.

This loss was such a good reminder to me to call the important people in my life and tell them what they mean to me. I feel fortunate that my final conversation with my dear Jeanie was filled with words of love.

One week later at 2 p.m., I arrived at her daughter's business, Jumpin' Janet's bar, where she choreographed a beautiful send-off for her beloved mother. The parking lot was packed, and every side street was lined with cars.

I walked into the crowded bar knowing only Janet. I glanced around and wondered who was who. I had heard so many tales about Jeanie's friends and family. Who was Roy—her first true love? Who was Brenda—her other daughter? Where was Cassie—her neighbor? As expected, they knew as much about me as I knew about them.

Jeanie loved Toby Keith's song "Red Solo Cup," so each seat had a bright red cup. Her favorite drink was Diet Pepsi; each cup had a full can tucked inside. Even though Jeanie was diabetic, each night before sleep she ate a small bite of a Nutty Buddy. A pair of cellophane-wrapped wafers sat on top of each cup. Allergies plagued this woman, so she was always walking around with handfuls or rolls of toilet paper. When I recommended Kleenex, she rebuffed me, scoffing at the unnecessary expense. A roll of toilet paper served as the centerpiece on each table. At Christmas, she made at least 60 loaves of banana bread and gifted them to her friends. Janet used the family recipe, and each table had ample slices of this delicacy sitting on paper plates covered in Saran wrap.

The pastor said a few words, Janet read the obituary, and then they opened the microphone to the crowd. After about five heartwarming tales, I took my turn. Tears started rolling down my face as I told the crowd about the circumstances surrounding my final conversation with Jeanie. I also said, "I don't know any of your faces, but I know so much about most of you. While Jeanie was ornery as hell and may have jumped in your faces many times, when she retold the stories to me, they were filled with love and compassion. She loved you all so much. Since you probably know more than your fair share about me, let's unite and honor Jeanie by keeping those secrets secret."

After many more stories, we wrote final goodbyes to Jeanie on pink Post-It Notes and attached them to pink, white, and purple helium-filled balloons. We stood in the strip mall parking lot and released our balloons in unison as Lynyrd Skynyrd's "Free Bird" blared from a lone speaker. The balloons in flight reminded me of the smoke ascending into the sky at the cremation on Mother Ganges. Another stream of tears flowed in that beautiful moment of letting go.

It was the nicest service. It honored Jeanie perfectly. Death is part of a well-lived life. Thanks to Jeanie and her daughter Janet, I finally had a true celebration of a great life in my own country.

Yogi Life Cycle

At birth, we arrive without any needs or expectations. Moments after our first breath, we begin the life cycle of demanding, expecting, wanting, desiring, and needing. We cry for Mama, and we cry for food.

We come into this incarnation with an undeveloped body and intelligence. The first 20 years of our lives are spent as a period of physical growth and education. We physically mature, experience puberty, and become capable of reproduction. The mind accumulates knowledge through experience and schooling.

The next 20 years are defined as a period of experimentation and implementation of our education. We work, travel, read, have sex, raise children, and live through more good and bad experiences. During this period our physical body tends to peak as we reach maximum muscle capacity and bone density.

From age 40-60, most people realize that accumulating and hoarding lead to overabundance. The need to have more and be the center of attention is replaced with a need to share our wealth. This impulse may include offering financial resources, wisdom, or time to others.

The next stage of life is one of total renunciation. Being closer to the finish allows a shift in focus. We give freely and share often, without expectation.

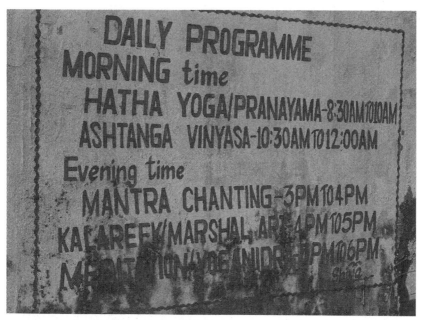

Simple Life

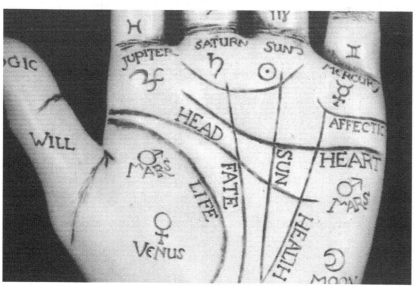

Rishikesh Street Art

Teaching My First Class

During the first two weeks of yoga training, a two-hour block was reserved every afternoon to practice breathing and asanas (yoga poses or postures). During the third week, Surinder changed the schedule and told us it was time to teach our own 40-minute class. He posted a sign-up sheet with 16 blank spaces. At two per afternoon, we would all have our chance to teach over the next eight afternoons. My German friend Ani took the liberty of signing me up for the number-one spot and she took the same afternoon. During dinner, she came up with a brilliant plan to combine our teaching in a manner where I would do 40 minutes of asana practice and she would lead a 40-minute shavasana (corpse pose) meditation. Nice try, Ani!

Instead of memorizing a bunch of postures, I spent my preparation time working on a story. I felt that the asanas would flow naturally if I just trusted my heart and let the story guide my class. We kept the same morning schedule, so on my day, I prepared to exit my room around 6 a.m. for our daily two-hour morning practice. When I opened the door, I found a note surrounded by a small gold elephant statue, a stick of incense, and two pieces of mango hard candy. The note, written on thick white paper, started with "Lovely Kurt" in bold black letters, underlined with a sparkly gold ink. The note read: "This little ganesha is for you. Ganesha is the lord of good fortune who provides fortune, success, and he protects us. He is the remover of obstacles and the lord of beginnings. You are such a wonderful and amazing soul. Enjoy your first class as a teacher!!"

At 3:45 p.m. I found myself sitting in front of Surinder, with 10 students on mats and six observing from bolsters placed along the back wall. I closed my eyes, inhaled deeply, and began chanting the "Om Sahana Vavatu" devotional peace mantra.

Om sahana vavatu
(Om, may God protect both teacher and student)
Saha nau bhunaktu
(May He nourish us together)
Saha viiryam karavaavahai
(May we work together with great energy)
Tejasvi nau-adhiitam-astu
(May our studying be effective)
Maa vidvissaavahai
(May there be no hate among us)
Om shanti, shanti, shanti
(Om peace, peace, peace [in three forms—
in me, nature, and the divine forces])

With all eyes focused on me, I began my story. Here it is:

"Try to imagine a huge castle surrounded by a large moat. Inside this immaculate building, almost everything is perfect. The food is exquisite and in unlimited supply. Custom furniture adorns every room, and beds are covered with thick Egyptian linens. Soothing music fills the halls, and the interior climate is always ideal. This castle is truly nirvana and is also known as the present moment in our lives.

"The only inhabitant that does not like being here is the Ego. Unfortunately, this one demands chronic attention. It has no purpose or source of contentment in the present moment. It suffocates inside and becomes powerless. For survival, it constantly cries and begs to go outside, across the moat, and into the promised land.

"The ego thrives in two spots across the moat. One, filled with regret, is the past. The other, specializing in anxiety and uncertainty, is known as the future.

"We each possess our own exquisite castle of the present moment. Unfortunately, we all cross the bridge and leave our utopias unwittingly. Rarely do we realize how far we have strayed from our castles.

"The best way to rectify our wanton ways is to acknowledge that we are not present and are instead bumbling around the useless fields of yesterday and tomorrow. The bridge back to the castle is always present, always free, and never demanding of anything. Breath is the bridge. No matter your time or place in life, you can always close your eyes and connect with your breath to take you home to the present moment.

"So today, please use this entire class to practice being present."

As expected, the asana portion of the class flowed naturally. It began with some seated warm-up postures, a series of sun salutations, a few standing poses, and a final shavasana. I felt a bit like a maestro, waving my words in front of the students and then watching their bodies contort in unison.

For the final portion of class, I encouraged my fellow students to bring their bolsters closer and sit to hear a final story:

"There is nothing wrong with our tendency to dive into our past. It is human and natural. Unfortunately, most of the time we are attracted to the darkness of yesterday and end up feeling depressed from actions or events that cannot be changed. It is like watching the same movie over and over, then being surprised that the ending is still the same. Yesterday's mistakes become nothing more than a hurtful whip we use to flog ourselves today. The best way to use the past is to go in, become aware that we are there, learn something, and quickly come back to the castle.

"Worry about the future is almost as worthless as swimming in the past. This does not mean we should all visit Vegas and put our life savings on red 21. Practical planning for food, shelter, and healthy living are necessities of life. The cancer of worry spreads when we allow the mind to believe that future events are real or likely to become fact. This 'fortune telling' ability creates ridiculous levels of fear and anxiety. If predicting the future was your actual career, you would have been fired a long time ago. When fretting about tomorrow, recognize this worry as a signal to use the breath as a bridge back to the present moment. Just as in yoga, this intention does not come naturally and only becomes easier with practice."

For the next week, my classmates each taught a class. Prior to their teaching, I had drifted into my future and thought, "This is kind of a bummer. Why are we being subjected to rookie teachers when we have Surinder?" This assumption proved to be another of my brilliant false prophesies.

By this time in the training, we had become a unified family. By sharing our personal visions of class, we were able to expose an intimate slice of ourselves that was not easily revealed through our daily interactions.

Marco from Portugal began his class by eloquently strumming the notes to Paul Simon's "The Sound of Silence" on an acoustic guitar. The words "Save Our Oceans" blazed across the chest of his green T-shirt. He began the lesson by telling his own story.

"It makes me angry," he said, "that our oceans are being polluted with chemicals and plastic. It makes me sad that this beautiful Ganges River has become one of the most polluted bodies of water in the world. The largest composition of my body is water. The same water that flows on these banks and eventually into the oceans. I will start to purify the world by making sure my own water is not tainted with impure actions or polluted by toxic thoughts."

Observing my fellow students exposing their souls without fear of judgment became another unexpected gift on this path.

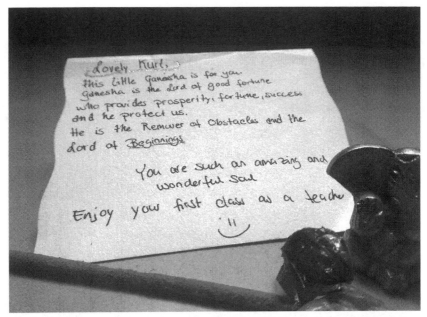

The Note

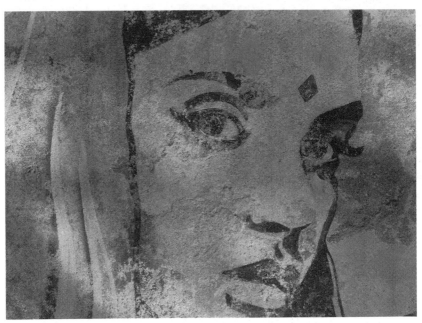

Rishikesh Street Art

Graduation

Our last day of the teacher-training program began like the previous sessions with a morning asana and pranayama practice. While we enjoyed our final breakfast together, Surinder taught the community drop-in class. At noon we gathered in the space where it all had begun a month ago.

A dining table filled about half of the room. Sixteen chairs surrounded a massive wood table with a 4-inch thick top. The other end of the room held a built-in couch that matched the rectangular shape of the space. Large beige cushions made this area a perfect place to lounge. A knee-high table served as a comforting place to rest the feet.

On our last day, Surinder and the three teachers sat at the base of the dining table while the entire class scrunched together in the couch area. Surinder kicked off the session by saying, "There is never an ending. Life and death are just a series of transitions. Do not be saddened by this ending. Instead, accept it as another new beginning."

He asked how many of the students had been to Rishikesh on previous trips. About half of the class members raised their hands. He then asked how many people really felt at home in this holy city. We all raised our hands. Unsurprised, he explained that many of the great yogis who had passed were still meditating in these mountains and our yogi souls were reuniting with our family.

After some congratulations he encouraged us to share some personal thoughts. At some point during the actual training, I think every person in the class had shed some tears. When it was my turn to speak, I said, "I lost a lot here. I lost some weight, some fear, and some bad habits."

Without notice, the tears began pouring out of my eyes. I continued, "What I gained will go with me to the grave. I gained a family. I gained a path to lifetime peace. Thank you, thank you, thank you."

One by one, we were called to the front of the room to be awarded our Certificate of Completion for 200 hours of Hatha yoga teacher training.

Surinder closed the ceremony with some simple words. He said, "Never stop being a student of yoga or of life. There will be times when your own ego will flatter you. Use that as your cue to be grateful and as a reminder to keep learning."

A few of my fellow students left on that same afternoon to return to their homes. With empty rooms in the yoga shala, the building felt like it had lost its soul.

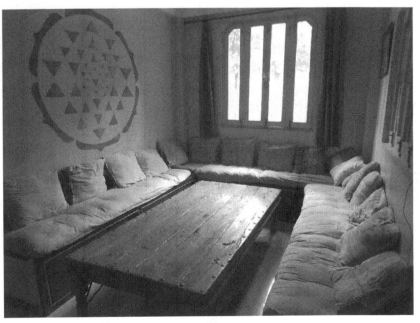

Rest Area

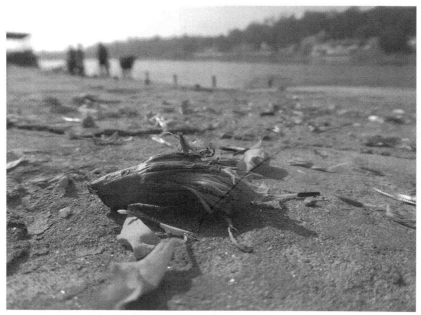

New Beginnings

Yoga Then and Now

When I look back at each decade of my life, I usually end up scratching my head and wondering, how could I have been so naive at each zero birthday? At 20, I obviously knew everything and could party like a rock star. I was indestructible and unburdened with consequences. At 30, I mastered business and was likely to be a CEO of a major company. At 40, I licked alcoholism and waded into international travel with visions of being the next Walter Mitty. At 50, I dabbled with Dharma.

Today, when my confidence grows in any endeavor, I remind myself that at my next zero birthday, my rear-view mirror will likely be filled with ignorance. Confidence is the warning light to immediately suppress my ego and open myself up to remaining a perpetual student.

The same cycle repeated itself in my past six years of yoga practice. In the moment, I always felt pretty good about my yoga practice. Looking back later on, I could see myself as a novice yogi. I now understand why they call yoga a "practice," because it can never be perfect, but always growing and changing. There is no endzone in which to score a touchdown.

On my first trip to India, my initial practice began with Iyengar yoga. This type of practice involves strict attention to detail and precision in each asana. My teacher, Ashish, had an uncanny ability to cause pain to dissipate with minor adjustments to each pose. Before this class, my lower back would always feel an extra burden in Warrior One. Ashish taught me how to position my hips in a manner that not only made the pose painless, but also added much-needed strength and confidence.

All of these experiences eventually led me to Surinder Singh and Hatha yoga. Hatha involves all the traditional asanas combined with a pranayama breathing practice. Most of the poses are held for longer periods of time and involve strength. The purpose of each Hatha session is to calm the soul to peacefully prepare the mind and body for a deeper spiritual practice.

Hatha literally means "force." One day Surinder asked, "Can anyone tell me why the Hindus always use coconut as an offering during religious rituals at the temples?" The question remained unanswered, so he continued. "The coconut, just like the ego, has a very hard shell. By using force, we crack the rough exterior and discover an interior that is soft and sweet. Break your shells and allow divine nectar to bring wisdom to your lives."

One day during a shavasana, Surinder told us a story about surface-level distractions. He said, "If you live life in an untethered manner, then you will be like a tiny buoy floating helplessly in the ocean. You will rise and fall with each disturbance. A constant flow of up and down. A problem happens, and you react." Looking deeply into our eyes he continued, "A better life exists well below the surface but requires a grounding force. It may be God, Spirit, the Universe, or even your yoga practice."

My initial foray into yoga was to firm my ass. Surinder taught me that yoga is much more about extracting my head from that same location.

He taught me how to take yoga off the mat and into my life. It was always by finding calmness, stillness, and inner peace.

Through this discovery process, my yoga has moved well beyond a physical practice. There are obvious physical benefits such as improved flexibility, balance, and strength. But these are minor intersections along a major highway to spiritual happiness.

When I practice yoga today, my eyes are closed 90% of the time, and I am mostly oblivious to my external surroundings. My focus is inward and on the breath: a far cry from my days of enjoying hot yoga mostly to enjoy the proximity of hot women. I now find good souls much more attractive than well-rounded bodies.

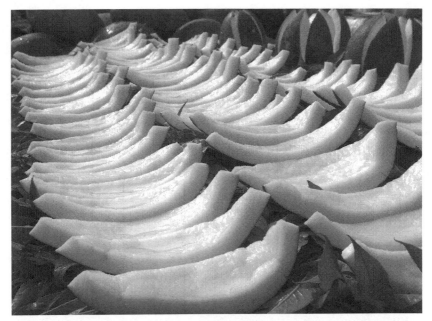

Street Cart Offerings

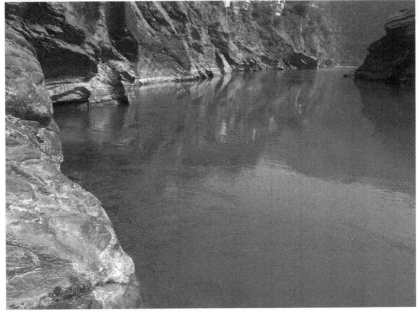

Stillness

Last Day

Sophie and I were the last two students to stay the night at Surinder's yoga shala. Most of the others had left the country. Some were still in Rishikesh at various guesthouses. I woke early with plans to see a few people. My first stop was The Juice House to have breakfast with Vishvas.

Prior to leaving my room, I prepared a handwritten card. I wanted him to know how much I appreciated his friendship, how much I admired his adherence to high moral standards, and how much I enjoyed his contagious positive outlook on life. I included some cash with the hope it would make his life a bit smoother.

We met at The Juice House around 8 a.m., and he made me a breakfast of muesli, fruit salad, and curd. He also made my favorite drink, "I Love Rishikesh," which included pomegranate, grapes, cinnamon, pineapple, mint, and cardamom. After I had eaten a few bites, he grinned and asked, "Does your breakfast taste different today?"

I answered, "It does, but I cannot figure it out. What is different?"

He said, "Coconut milk is special. For your last day, I used this instead of the curd."

I gave him the card and asked him to open it the next day when he was alone. He smiled and handed me a card that he too had written prior to our breakfast meeting. Lord Shiva was on the cover, and Vishvas' words were of gratitude for our friendship. I tried to pay for the meal on the way out and he said, "Don't be silly on your final day. Enjoy!"

With a full stomach and a big smile, I continued down the street with intention to walk through Parmarth for a last but not permanent goodbye. As I passed the Jai Neelkanth Restaurant, Arpit, like a sentry, was at the street-side cashier's stand. With a big grin he said, "So Mr. Kurt, this is in fact your final day in Rishikesh. Am I correct?"

"Yes," I replied. "It has been wonderful and thank you for giving me so much of your time on this visit. I will look forward to seeing you next year."

With a cagey smile, he reached under the counter and lifted a clear bag filled with several items wrapped in newspaper. He said, "My mom did not want you to leave India without proper food, so she made this food for your long flight home." After a hug of thanks, I humbly walked the last block back to Parmarth.

The Parmarth grounds were sacred to me. There was an amazing feeling of positive energy each time my feet touched the property. The chronic chaos of India seemed to melt away in the ashram.

I walked out the back entrance and toward one of my favorite streets. The play of light and shadow on this particular road always made for great photo shoots. It was also the path I took to my very first Indian yoga class. As I circled back to the main road, my friend Raj was serving chai at his new tea stand. He said, "When are you going home?"

"Today," I said.

"You cannot leave without my art," he insisted.

He began to unwrap a large scroll of finished paintings. Thumbing through them, he stopped on a large face of a golden Buddha and said, "This is the one that needs to go home with you." He quickly wrapped it in newspaper and secured the ends with duct tape. "This is my gift to you."

However, as soon as the painting was in my hands, he began negotiating the price. I laughed, remembering the time he asked me to pay his rent. I figured the word "gift" meant something different to Raj, but truly, his art was a gift, no matter the cost. Like the other piece I had already hung in my bedroom in Boise, this painting would also find its home in my home. I gifted Raj many rupees in return.

Then, after a huge hug, I began the short walk to Narayan's store for my final chai and a photo shoot. On the first day of this trip, I had given him a copy of my Camino book, *A Million Steps*. He wanted a photograph with the two of us by the river holding the book. I sat on my normal plywood seat as he shook his head back and forth—in amazement, we discussed how fast time passes. Bablu served us chai and a roll of coconut biscuits. At the appropriate time, Narayan looked at me and said, "I need to change clothes. I only have one outfit, and I wear it to every wedding. It is 20 years old, but it is my best." Humbled by his words, I waited for him to reemerge in black pants that matched his formal black top. He had arranged for his friend to snap pictures and we took at least 30 shots. He insisted on photos with the River Ganges as background, glasses on and glasses off; with the ghat steps as background, glasses on and glasses off. With another big hug, I said goodbye to my dear friend Narayan.

Not sure what to do with the rest of the time, I began to wander. Halfway across the Ram Jhula Bridge, I glanced downstream toward the cremation grounds. There was no activity, so I decided to walk down there and spend a few moments paying silent respect to the area. I sat on a random rock and just watched the powerful river dance.

Suddenly, four men walked past me with large pieces of wood on their shoulders. I turned my head and saw another group of eight men with their right arms wrapped around more wood balanced on their shoulders. They all deposited the wood in a pile by the water. The stream of men continued for about 15 minutes. Some carried material as large as railroad ties, others had smaller sticks, and a few had bundles of fire-starting brush. Like craftsman, they skillfully pulled pieces from the pile and began to construct a pyre with a perfectly flat surface. The work stopped, and they all looked up at the path leading to the river.

Four men held their respective corners of the homemade gurney. On top lay a body, covered in a white shroud and draped with garlands of marigolds. The group made its way to the river. Lowering the gurney to the ground, they lifted the shroud alone and placed it on the structure. The men finished the construction of the pyre by covering the body with the remaining pile of wood. About 10 feet from the cremation site, the group of mourners started a small fire and conducted a ceremony. One young man, probably the eldest son, then lit a torch from the ceremonial fire. With the torch, he ignited his father's cremation pyre.

As I sat on a large boulder, near where I viewed my first cremation, I began to absorb the full circle of my experience on this site. The first time, I witnessed the ceremony from the midpoint to the end. This time I witnessed it all from the raw beginning. Unlike my third-grade experience with my grandmother, this ceremony seemed like a natural and necessary part of dying.

As I approached the bridge to return to my guesthouse, I passed a small shop and literally bumped into Surinder. Of course the opportunity to say goodbye happened exactly in this manner. What's more, about a half a mile from the guesthouse, I stuck my head in the door of the Ayurvedic Café and was not at all surprised to see Sona and Juan enjoying a meal. When I arrived at the yoga shala, the only pair of shoes on the shoe rack was my blue thongs. Sophie was walking out the door, and I hoisted her backpack onto her shoulders.

Later, I began my final walk to say goodbye to Mother Ganga. Halfway to the river, a white-haired man dressed in traditional orange pulled up on his scooter, stopped to look at me, and said, "Who are you and what are you doing here?"

I told him about being a student of Surinder and how much I loved Rishikesh. He pointed over my shoulder and said, "That is my ashram, please come and say hi on your next visit." He revved the engine and took off down the road.

I arrived at the river and saw my flower pal, Ardul. Of course, I had to buy a puja bowl to send down the river. I asked Ganga for safe travels back to my home.

My final goodbye goal in Rishikesh was to spend some time on a specific rock where I had enjoyed meditation. From afar, I saw someone already sitting there. When I got closer, I realized it was my new white-haired scooter friend. We sat and meditated together.

At the end, he looked at me and said, "It will be most interesting to finish this conversation next year."

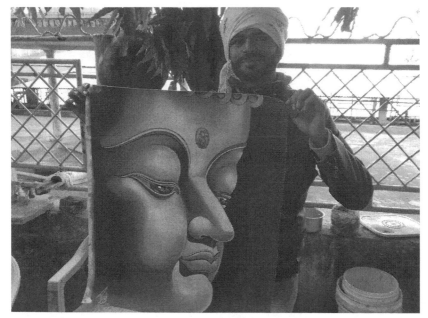

Raj

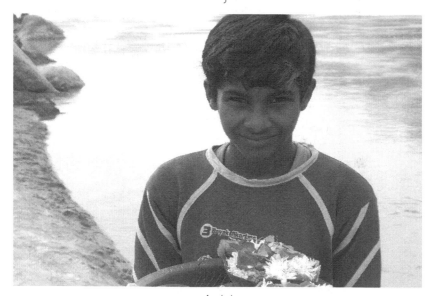

Ardul

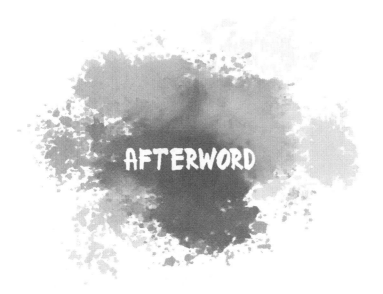

AFTERWORD

Yoga Back Home

About halfway through our teacher training, I let my mind slip into the future with questions of where and how I would practice yoga at home. I still planned to attend some hot yoga classes but needed space for a pure Hatha practice. I had tried many local instructors but had trouble finding a teacher who went slowly, held long poses, and could synchronize with my breath. Nothing was more frustrating than to hear a teacher tell me to follow my breath and then call out the movements in a manner likely to cause hyperventilation.

During my yoga teacher-training course, the solution found its way into my head and heart.

My Boise home has three bedrooms. At this point, I had lived in this home for 27 years and would wager that I had been in the third bedroom about once a year.

Ten years ago, I bought a new couch for my living room and did not have any use for the old furniture. I decided to put it into the unused bedroom with the hope of making it a serene environment for reading and relaxing. Well, over the next 10 years, I never once sat on that old couch. From Surinder's yoga shala, I decided to give the furniture to a friend and replace the carpet with flooring that would be conducive to a home yoga studio.

The room has three walls that begin to make a perfect square until the fourth wall intersects at a 45-degree angle to create a unique shape. The room's window and walls were barren. An antique mirror from my deceased father's home leaned against one wall.

Thoughts of this oak-framed mirror triggered another story that Surinder had shared during one of his satsung sessions. He said, "What do you see when you look in the mirror? Most see something that looks good or something that needs to be repaired. In life, no one teaches anyone how to interpret their own reflection. Meditation is shining a mirror on the inside. Unlike the exterior, there is never anything to fix because the divine is inside of everyone, and that is total perfection. Forget your external and teach yourself how to reflect from your unblemished interior."

From India, I dipped into my Western ways and did some shopping through my Amazon account. I bought two blue round bolsters with the *om* symbol embroidered on the ends. I bought four blue foam blocks, a few straps, and a pad for my aging knees.

The day after I returned home, Robby from Idaho Floor Supply came to my house to help me choose a floor. "I would like to put some hardwood in here," I told him.

"Good for you," he replied, "but you will need to hire someone else to ruin this room. If you want to use me, then you need a cork floor."

A week later his crew installed a cork floor in my yoga room. I had the mirror raised off the floor and permanently attached to the wall. A shelf below the mirror became home to a small singing bowl. Next to the bowl I placed a set of Tibetan tingsha chimes that I had purchased the prior year. An 8-inch leather cord held the heavy gold cymbals in place for the perfect, gentle collision to create a soothing sound.

Lacking additional decorating skills, I asked a friend from the gym to take over and keep the space open and free of clutter. She added some long sheer curtains that flowed from a black iron rod. I framed and hung the Gold Buddha painting that Raj "gave" me on my last day in Rishikesh.

A friend's daughter finished the room by painting a rainbow-colored *om* symbol on another wall. The wall painting is about 5 by 5 feet, with a large cloudlike circle surrounding the symbol. Music notes and two birds drift toward the sky.

Because the mirror hangs on the 45-degree wall, I find it hard to see external reflections in my home studio. The mirror's presence reminds me of my father and the need to reflect from within. The gifted painting had a purpose. The moment that Raj gave it to me, I knew his Golden Buddha would be part of my home yoga scene. The *om* wall keeps me constantly grounded and reminds me of my infinite nature.

If I were to actually think of my house as a human body, the downstairs location of this small room could easily be considered the heart. My home now beats from within.

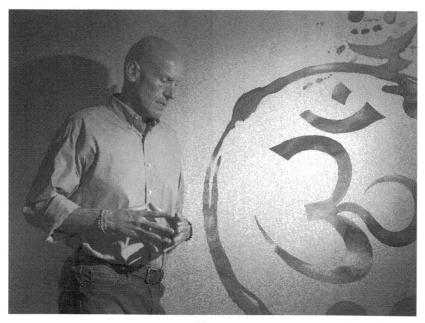

Home

Stay in Touch

I would love to speak at your local yoga studio, yoga retreat, corporate meeting, or wellness event. I have developed an hour-long presentation to share stories and photos from my yoga travels throughout the world. I am also available to teach Hatha yoga classes at these events. Booking information is available at my website (see below).

Feel free to connect on my personal Facebook page to keep up with my recent travels or visit the Kurt Koontz Author/Speaker page for daily inspirational messages and information on upcoming events.

I offer a free subscription to my weekly blog posts. An extensive library of previous stories will take you around the world several times. Please visit my website for more information.

If you would like to sell this book at your yoga studio, contact me for special pricing and promotional materials.

Please consider writing a review for this book on Amazon.

I personally respond to all phone calls, emails, and social media messages. If you feel the urge, reach out, and we will connect!

My Cell Phone: (208) 345-6421
Email: k@kurtkoontz.com
Website: www.kurtkoontz.com

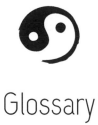

Glossary

asanas – yoga postures or positions.

bindi – a decorative mark worn in the middle of the forehead, representing the third eye of wisdom in Hinduism.

ghee – clarified butter used in cooking and religious rituals.

ganesha – elephant-headed Hindu deity. The god of beginnings, success, and wisdom.

Hatha yoga – yoga training that is openly available to anyone. Includes both physical poses and breath training.

havan – a religious offering made into fire.

Iyengar yoga – a form of Hatha yoga that emphasizes detail, precision, and alignment.

mantra – a sacred sound, syllable, word, or group of words.

mudra – a ritual gesture in Hinduism and Buddhism.

namaskar mudra – palms of hands pressed together at the chest to show respect and devotion.

Om – sacred sound and symbol in the Hindu religion.

prana – life force.

pranayama – breath training to enhance life force.

puja – a ritual to express honor, worship, and devotion.

santsang – a spiritual discourse or sacred gathering.

shavasana – "corpse" pose usually done at end of yoga practice, when practitioners lie on their backs with legs and hands relaxed at their sides.

swasti – well-being or welcome.

Vinyasa yoga – a form of yoga that emphasizes breath and movement flowing from one pose to the next.

Yin yoga – a slow-paced form of yoga that holds positions for long periods.

yoga shala – yoga studio.

yogi – a practitioner of yoga.

Acknowledgments

My content editor, Jeanette Germain, spent over 100 hours working on this book. I know it was in her mind and heart for much longer, but thankfully she did not bill me for the extra mountain of time.

Our professional relationship began in 2012 with *A Million Steps* and quickly blossomed into a deep friendship. With this book, she encouraged me to write short stories without any worry about how they would connect. I delivered a massive, unorganized, rambling group of tales, and she figured out how to stitch them together. At one point, she printed the first page of each story, laid the pages out on her office floor, and shuffled them into a narrative. Without her enormous contribution, there would be no *Practice* story quilt.

Jeanette happens to live a few blocks from my home. When we worked on the Camino book, we occasionally walked together along the nearby river to discuss our progress. For this book, she walked to my house for several face-to-face meetings. After the business, we practiced together in my home yoga studio. These are priceless memories.

Chris Trecani (www.3dogcreative.net) was also instrumental in helping me bring this book to you. After reading the manuscript, he designed and created several potential book covers. He took my thoughts and turned them into art. In addition, Chris uploaded book files to the various vendors. That task is also an art! He designed and maintains my website. If you need creative talent, I would highly recommend his services.

My copy editor, Courtney Harler (courtneyharler.wordpress.com), is new to this team. She was referred to me to me by a local superstar author.

Courtney lives in Las Vegas, so we did not have a chance to meet in person. Through many phone calls and emails, we also developed a nice friendship. I look forward to meeting her in person someday. It was nice to be able to write in my own voice knowing there was a professional backstop to prevent unintentional errors. If you are looking for professional services to complement your writing endeavors, stop shopping and hire Courtney.

Sean Johnson (www.seanjohnsonart.com) created the maps at the beginning of this book. He is a fellow Camino pilgrim. We met briefly during my first book tour and became Facebook friends. One day, he sent me a private message asking if he could draw a few of my Rishikesh photos. A few months later, two prints showed up on my doorstep. Who does that for a stranger? They hang in my home office, and I appreciate them daily.

Lastly, I would like to reach out to the entire yoga community. I have met some of the most astounding teachers through my travels, and every one of them has imprinted a bit of their soul into my personal practice. I cherish the camaraderie I have found with my fellow yogis from around the world.

Made in the USA
San Bernardino, CA
24 October 2018